THE HEALTHY

INDIAN DIET

How Traditional Foods of South Asia Help
Prevent Heart Disease, Diabetes and Cancer

WRITTEN BY RAJ R. PATEL, M.D.

RECIPES BY
HETAL JANNU AND
ANUJA BALASUBRAMANIAN

Inquiries should be addressed to:
Raj R. Patel, M.D.
PO Box 667234
Houston, Texas 77266
RajRPatelMD@gmail.com

First Edition
First Printing (June 2011)
Cataloguing-in-Publication Data
The Healthy Indian Diet by Raj R. Patel, Anuja Balasubramanian, and Hetal Jannu
p. cm.
Includes bibliographical references and index
ISBN-13: 978-1461122135
ISBN-10: 1461122139
1. Health & Fitness – Food and Diet.
2. Cooking – Indian Food.
3. Health & Fitness – Prevention.
Library of Congress shelving number pending
Dewey decimal number pending

Author's note. Although information herein is based on the author's extensive experience and knowledge, this book is not intended to be a substitute for care and counsel provided by medical professionals. All matters regarding your health require medical supervision. Neither the author nor the publisher shall be liable or responsible for any loss or damage allegedly arising from any information or suggestion in this book. Consult your physician before adopting advice in this book if you have any known or unknown medical condition.

Printed in the United States of America
by Sun Health Press, subsidiary of Surya Health, L.L.C.
at CreateSpace, L.L.C.

Cover Design by Anita Amit

TABLE OF CONTENTS

INTRODUCTION

Hippocrates, the ancient Greek physician known as the Father of Western Medicine, once said, "Let food be thy medicine." Indeed, for hundreds of years before and after him, physicians had little at their disposal besides food and other elements found in nature to treat disease. Millennia of experiments and observations on animals and people revealed to pre-modern healers what actually worked, and which plants, herbs and spices helped people recover their health and stay well. Unbeknownst to them, foods are made of molecules that interact with the molecules making up the human body. These interactions help or harm the body, just like medications.

WHY I WROTE A BOOK ON THE HEALTHY INDIAN DIET

In this book, I examine how food can be good medicine, especially in the context of chronic diseases that have grown to epidemic proportions both here and the world over. I focus on Indian foods, which, according to famous American and European doctors like Mehmut Oz, M.D., David Servan-Schreiber, M.D., and Dean Ornish, M.D, are very beneficial to human health. I initially found this position to be odd because, growing up as an Indian-American kid, I developed the impression that Indian food was bad for your health. This cognitive dissonance between what I knew growing up and this new perspective on Indian food compelled me to find out who, in fact, was right.

I also examined the latest published experiments and observations speaking on the relationship between diet and human health. The past couple years of this journey have bore some fruit, as the pieces have started to come together. I now realize that the *modern* Indian diet is indeed bad for you. It was surprising to learn exactly what in the modern Indian diet was bad: whereas I once thought the rash of heart

1

attacks among middle-aged men in my community was explained by eating a lot of *ghee*, I could see that thanks to new knowledge, it wasn't the *ghee* but actually refined grains, starchy vegetables, and sugar.

THE HEALTHY INDIAN DIET

The *traditional* Indian diet is what these famous doctors are actually referring to, and the foods in this diet in fact do the body a lot of good. Like the Mediterranean Diet, the most famous and well-studied of traditional diets, the traditional Indian diet is low on refined grains, starchy vegetables, and sugar. This means it is full of whole grains, leafy vegetables, and spices. Whereas other traditional diets from around the world are found to be good for people, what sets the Indian diet apart from the others is the presence of spices like turmeric and black pepper in everyday meals.

Spices also tie all regional diets of the Indian subcontinent together, just like olive oil and fatty fish tie all the various Mediterranean regional diets together. In the past decade or so, spices have been under the microscope lens of modern science, and many have been found to be astonishingly beneficial. The same is true of other elements of a traditional or *healthy* Indian diet. Unlike medications, spices and foods tend to have low, if any, adverse effects in most people, and no side effects whatsoever in those who are accustomed to eating them.

I have written this book for two reasons. One, I want to highlight what modern science tells us about how various foods help us stay healthy and improve our well-being, especially in the context of diseases such as obesity, heart disease, diabetes, and cancers. Two, I want to propose an alternative to the Mediterranean Diet based on the traditional cuisines of India, which includes many nutrient-dense whole foods. To give a compelling alternative, I have had to define what a healthy Indian diet means. I hope you find the concepts easy to grasp, that the evidence persuades you to my way of thinking on this issue, and that you allow for the elements of the healthy Indian diet to "be thy medicine."

How to Read This Book

Many pages of this book are devoted to the science of foods, how diets affect the development of chronic diseases, and what constitutes a *healthy* Indian diet. These sections can get quite technical, and I have written them for readers who are intellectually curious about how the body works and how the foods we eat every day influence our overall health. These pages also give credibility to the idea that the healthy Indian diet is indeed good for you.

However, if you want to know what constitutes a healthy Indian diet and then begin preparing meals that fit the profile, skip to Part II and begin reading from there. I intended to make this book practical, and I have included recipes at the end thanks to two wonderful women, Hetal and Anuja, who teach people how to make Indian dishes – many of them healthy.

There is a section toward the end of the book more specific to people from the Indian subcontinent. I started this project with this in mind: people all over the world are suffering from chronic diseases, but people of South Asian descent suffer them in greater numbers. Additionally, I have included a Glossary to help readers with certain terms that I have elected to use the Hindi word for, such as *haldi* (turmeric powder).

Diet, Not Dieting

Before going on, I want to make a clear distinction between "diet" and "dieting." This book focuses on a daily diet or pattern of foods, leaving you to pick and choose which elements you want to emphasize based on your (and your family's) tastes. I do not get specific about how much of something to eat, or indeed how often. It is useful to think of the advice here as more like guidelines than fixed rules.

If you wish to follow a prescription of certain foods in specific amounts for a more specific goal, such as losing weight or gaining muscle, then this is not the book for you. While you can emphasize elements of the healthy Indian diet to help lose weight, I focus on

3

describing basic elements of Indian foods that compel readers to adhere to the diet in the long-term, motivated by the knowledge that the diet is healthy, and because the diet is tasty.

My approach emphasizes that changing your diet to something healthier, whether you already eat Indian food or not, is difficult. So rather than trying to switch overnight, I hope you aim to change your diet gradually. For example, don't throw out the white rice immediately and replace it with brown rice. Instead, cook brown rice two or three nights a week, substituting meals where you have white rice. After some weeks, if you find you like the taste of brown rice, or feel it is important to switch, then keep going.

Fortunately, this kind of diet – a change in the patterns of foods you eat – is easier to stick with. After all, today's dishes have come from hundreds of years of cooking various combinations of foods, and they have made it this far because they taste good and provide the body with the nutrition it needs.

THIS IS NOT AYURVEDA

If you want to learn about *Ayurveda*, the Indian tradition of health and healing, please refer to a book based on that specific subject, not this book. For the uninitiated reader, *Ayurveda* is a millennia-old metaphysical system based on how five elements – fire, water, earth, air, and ether – combine to make the seven constituent elements of the human body. Ayurvedic practitioners aim to maintain the balance between these seven constituents to keep a person healthy. The principal way of maintaining this balance is by eating foods according to your strongest elemental energy, either *vata*, *pitta*, or *kapha*. Adhering to this means restricting certain foods.

Ayurveda is not a relic of the past, as it is taught in medical schools and practiced professionally in India to this day. Millions of Indians prefer to visit an Ayurvedic physician rather than a physician trained in the Western mold, seeking a traditional healing method over new technology. Many people in the West who are disenchanted with modern medicine also seek out Ayurvedic physicians. All of this keeps the body of knowledge alive and well.

Despite acknowledging that there is some merit in the *Ayurveda* system, this book does not talk about a healthy Indian diet in that context. I have been unable find any evidence in medical literature to support the idea that one should eat according to one's fundamental energy to maintain good health. This is not to say that science will not one day prove that this is the optimal way to eat. However, I have to go by the evidence present today.

Furthermore, I have written this book to let you, the reader living in the modern world with access to a variety of foods unimaginable even a decade ago, pick and choose and craft your own version of the healthy Indian diet.

THE POWER OF THE HEALTHY INDIAN DIET

Once upon a time, when a child of South Asian descent fell sick with a cold or sore throat, his mother gave him a concoction made of turmeric powder – and it worked! This isn't really once upon a time. Indian mothers still give their children, whether they are in a big American city or a tiny village in India, a variation turmeric-based concoction when they fall ill.

As a grown man who is a physician by training and skeptical of alternative medicine, I still take that "potion" of warmed-up milk plus a teaspoon of turmeric powder and a pinch of salt when I get a cold or sore throat. Though this isn't a proven remedy in medical literature, it has always worked for me. I am sure because it is a potion of sorts and tastes like medicine (i.e., awful), it exerts a certain placebo effect, by which I mean it may not treat the illness at all. No matter, I definitely *feel* like it does.

Thanks to my recent reading of the scientific literature, I now know that turmeric powder has anti-bacterial and anti-inflammatory properties. In this context, my observation that a bad sore throat goes away within a day after drinking this stuff – and similar observations by others – likely provides an underlying explanation. And now, modern science has begun to show that turmeric powder – a universal ingredient in Indian cooking – can help your body fight cancers.

IS THE HOLY GRAIL IN THE INDIAN DIET?

Researchers at M.D. Anderson Cancer Center in Houston have demonstrated that curcumin, the bioactive molecule in turmeric powder, prevents cancer cells from growing. Chemotherapies also prevent cancer cells from growing, but there is a key difference. Chemotherapies have significant side effects because they also attack the body's normal cells. Curcumin does not. Turmeric powder, like any food people eat, has no side effects in small amounts generally speaking (as it is had in Indian dishes). Curcumin causes at most gastrointestinal discomfort in large and purified amounts.

In dramatic fashion, researchers at John Hopkins have shown what curcumin can do in living people. Five patients with a rare form of colon cancer called Familial Adenomatous Polyposis (FAP)[i] enrolled in a small clinical trial where they took 480 mg of curcumin and 20 mg of quercetin (a phytonutrient found in onions) three times a day for six months. They took no other medication for FAP.[1]

Remarkably, 60% of each patient's pre-cancerous polpys vanished! The remaining polpys shrunk to half their original size on average. Importantly, there were no toxic effects from the curcumin or the quercetin.

Celexocib, a COX-2 inhibitor medication marketed as Celebrex, has a similar effect on those polyps. In another trial of 15 FAP patients taking 400 mg of celexocib twice a day for six months, 30% of a patient's polyps were gone on average.[2] The remaining polyps shrunk from their original size by about a third. But taking celexocib comes with a price – an increased risk of heart attacks. This is why the FDA advises physicians to use caution when prescribing it.

Side effects are a vexing issue for patients and their doctors, and not just side effects from cancer-targeted medications. Commonly taken pills cause side effects that make many people stop taking them. Beta blockers (like metoprolol), which is used for treating blood pressure, can cause severe fatigue, and statins (like atorvastatin), used to regulate cholesterol levels, can cause muscle inflammation. Foods, in particular those foods that people are accustomed to eating as part of traditional diets, do not cause such severe side effects. What if food could help prevent, or even treat, high blood pressure and bad cholesterol levels?

---

[i] People with this disease have hundreds of polpys, essentially pre-cancerous lesions, and will develop cancer by age 40 if they are left untreated.

Well, food can. Many spices and herbs like black pepper and garlic reduce the detrimental effects of inflammation, a process linked to cancers and heart disease. Whole foods in a *traditional* diet, like *channa* (chickpeas) and brown rice, prevent spikes in the hormone insulin and thus reduce the risk of obesity and diabetes. Cutting down on salt lowers high blood pressure, the leading risk factor for strokes. In short, eating a healthy Indian diet almost daily will help you reduce the risk of developing chronic diseases with devastating complications, and it will help you maintain your general well-being.

MODERN LIGHT ON INDIAN FOOD

Experts in human health are starting to recognize the power of the increasingly popular healthy Indian diet. The findings on turmeric powder from M.D. Anderson Cancer Center likely inspired Dr. David Servan-Schreiber, a psychiatrist and researcher who survived brain cancer, to write that the Indian diet (along with the Mediterranean and Asian diets) is an anti-cancer diet. Dr. Dean Ornish, a preventive cardiologist who defied medical dogma by showing that the narrowing of coronary arteries could be reversed by lifestyle changes alone, believes in the power of Indian food.

He described dishes and beverages he likes in "The Healing Secrets of Food: A Practical Guide for Nourishing Body, Mind, and Soul," but he did not define the elements of a healthy Indian diet. Even Dr. Mehmut Oz, the heart surgeon who is now the most popular physician in the U.S., has heaped praise on traditional Indian food on his television show.

Now that "Let's go get some Indian food" is a popular suggestion on a weekend night among Americans from all walks of life, and as more experts trumpet how healthy the Indian diet seems to be, more Western researchers are investigating these claims. This is nothing new, as there are findings from decades of research conducted on Indian diets in India that support its health benefits. It may be hard to believe, but even during the colonial era, physicians found evidence of how people developed disease when they abandoned their traditional diet for a modern one.

I believe science will ultimately show that much in the traditional Indian diet is good for you, just as science has done for the traditional Mediterranean diet. This book, I hope, will shed light on the power of the Indian diet based on what scientists are beginning to substantiate and on what we have already known in the collective consciousness for years.

Knowledge is power, and after you finish reading this book, you will know what constitutes a healthy diet, especially what constitutes a healthy Indian diet, and be better able to draw from the power found in a healthy Indian diet. But before I define the elements, I want to make a clear case for why it is important to start adopting elements of a healthy Indian diet today.

PART I
THE SCIENCE
OF CHRONIC
DISEASES AND
FOOD BASICS

THE EPIDEMIC OF CHRONIC DISEASE

To have our fist idea of things we must see those things. To have an idea about natural phenomenon we must, first of all, observe it. The mind of man cannot conceive an effect without a cause so that the sight of a phenomena always awakens an idea of causation. All human knowledge is limited from working back from observed effects to their causes.

– Claude Bernard

THE STORY OF A BRITISH PHYSICIAN WHO FOUND THE ROOTS OF CHRONIC DISEASES IN COLONIAL INDIA

Robert McCarrison, M.D. landed on the shores of India in 1901. He had finished his medical training in Belfast only months before and, like many fellow Irishmen, embarked to the British Raj to further his career. At the ripe age of 23, McCarrison was posted in the mountainous Northern Frontiers to be a medical officer for a regiment of Indian sepoys. He would spend the better part of three decades in India, pioneering research in areas where nutrition, diet, and health intersect. He then retired to Oxford, was knighted, and was elevated to the rank of the King's Honourable Physician.

However, in 1901, McCarrison was busy caring for troops guarding the Himalayan border as a junior physician. For the next dozen years, he was thus preoccupied but still found time to record his observations on the Hunza diet and their overall health. The good health enjoyed by the Hunza left an impression on the young doctor, and he compared their diet to the diets of surrounding tribes and villages. After finding a high incidence of thyroid goiter in some Himalayan villages, he began performing simple experiments on rats, other animals, and eventually people, including himself, to discover the reason.

12

The young doctor learned that the people who suffered goiter disease ate a diet lacking in iodine. Worse, iodine deficiencies led to cretinism, a devastating childhood disease that impairs normal development. Cretin children were found to be born to mothers who did not have enough iodine in their food.[ii] After gaining worldwide acclaim for his discoveries, McCarrison's superiors allowed him to spend most of his time conducting nutrition research after 1913.

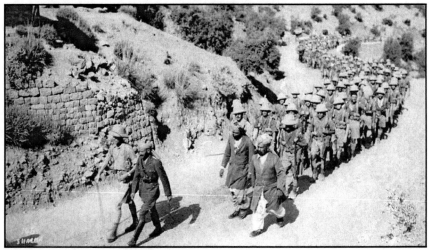

Figure 1: British and Indian soldiers marching. (Photo used under Creative Commons from Northampton Museum.)

For the next several years, McCarrison traveled around British India and found regions where a particular disease was rampart, then sat down to figure out what deficiency was causing the disease. He found a high incidence of beriberi, a debilitating disease of the heart, muscles, nerves, and intestines among villagers near Bombay. He worked out that beriberi was caused by a deficiency of thiamine (vitamin B1). It is here that he began linking disease to the modernization of diet. In his 1924 paper on beriberi, McCarrison explained that thiamine deficiency was caused by the local rice being "decorticated."[3]

In other words, rice grains were so refined that their germ and

---

[ii] McCarrison's discovery of the role of iodine deficiency and thyroid diseases eventually led to our table salt being fortified with iodine.

bran, where the nutrition and fiber resides, were taken out, leaving only the starch-rich endosperm – in other words, white rice. Refined rice became popular after people recognized that it doesn't rot as quickly as whole grain rice, and was thus easier to sell and store. The villagers, who for generations had eaten whole grain rice that was not milled, were now eating white rice lacking critical vitamins like thiamine and fiber and contributing to a quickly usable form of energy. McCarrison's travels, observations, and experiments led him to form an underlying explanation for chronic diseases, including diabetes, heart disease, and even tuberculosis, that sounds astonishingly contemporary: "The extensive use of vitamin-poor white flour and [the] inordinate use of vitamin-less sugar."[4]

In 1918, McCarrison began a small lab in Coonoor in the pleasant Nilgiri Hills of Tamil Nadu. Ten years later, he became the Director of Nutritional Research in India, and he spent most of his life there until he retired conducting nutrition experiments.[iii] It was during this tenure that he performed one of his more famous experiments. His team divided 1,200 albino rats into eight groups and fed each group a different regional Indian diet. He found that the Punjabi Sikh diet, resembling in many ways the Hunza diet that had impressed him early in his career, kept the rats the healthiest, leanest, and best prepared against infections. McCarrison elaborated on the diet in a 1936 lecture.

> In general the races of northern India are wheat-eaters, though they make use also of certain other whole cereal grains. Now the biological value of the proteins of whole wheat is relatively high; and the wheat is eaten whole, after being freshly ground into a coarse flour (atta) and made into cakes called chapattis. It thus preserves all the nutrients with which Nature has endowed it, particularly its proteins, its vitamins and its mineral salts. The second most important ingredient of their diet is milk, and the products of milk (clarified butter or ghee, curds, buttermilk); the third is dhal (pulse); the fourth, vegetables and fruit. Some eat meat sparingly, if at all; others, such as the Pathans, use it in considerable quantity. Their

---

[iii] This lab would become India's National Institute of Nutrition, now based in Hyderabad.

food thus contains – when they can get the food they want, which they do not always do – all elements and complexes needed for normal nutrition (with the possible exception of iodine in some Himalayan regions) and abundance of those things that matter from the point of view of the structural and functional efficiency of the body.[5]

According to McCarrison's experiments on the diets of British India, the Sikhs' traditional diet was the best in terms of health. It was based on coarsely ground wheat, milk and fermented dairies, *dals*, vegetables, fruit, and even meat. In his view, the worst diet for health was that of the "rice-eaters of the south and east of India." The Madrassi diet, as he called it, was "excessively rich in carbohydrates, and [there was] deficiency of protein, mineral salts and vitamins."

His team recorded "high infant mortality, poor growth, disease of various kinds and premature death" among the rats fed the Madrassi diet, and McCarrison observed the same kinds of diseases affecting people in South India who ate this kind of diet.[6] McCarrison blamed the effects of the Madrassi diet largely on rice, which wasn't prevalent in the Sikh diet, because it was the poorest grain in regard to nutrition.

Worse than rice were refined grains of any kind. Production and the sale of Indian foods became increasingly industrialized during the British Raj. Practices like heavy refining of grains to give them longer shelf lives became more common, and McCarrison didn't like what he was seeing. He said:

> I have little patience with those who would have us believe that 'white flour' is as good an article of diet as 'whole wheat flour'. White flour, when used as the staple article of diet, [cause people] to build up their dietaries with a staple of relatively low nutritive value.[7]

When McCarrison moved to Oxford, England in 1935 after decades of research that illuminated connections between what people ate and their overall health, he was brimming with ideas. Western governments took his findings, replicated by others, and began requiring manufacturers to fortify foods with vitamins to prevent against deficiencies. While his work on diseases of single nutritional deficiencies was widely read and followed, his philosophy of using whole foods as medicine was mostly ignored. In his later years, he began to emphasize that people should eat foods as they are found in nature. But this idea and his conclusions on nutrient-dense traditional Indian diets ideal for human health have been largely forgotten.

The era of antibiotics had arrived, and soon factories were producing insulin. These miracles made doctors and researchers worship at the altar of technologies that could treat and even cure disease. They thus became more interested in the treatment of disease rather than in their prevention, which was McCarrison's passionate response to fighting illness. In his later years, McCarrison deplored the increasing consumption of refined white flour and the substitution of canned, preserved and artificially sweetened products for fresh, natural, whole foods in the U.K. and America. The epidemics of chronic diseases that took root in the West were sadly a result of those trends.

THE GLOBAL EPIDEMIC OF OBESITY AND THE MODERNIZATION OF DIETS

No longer is it shocking to read that chronic diseases – namely obesity, diabetes, coronary heart disease, and many cancers – have become so common in modern societies that health experts refer to them using the word "epidemic." And it may be not too shocking to learn that the rising rates of heart disease and diabetes, which have been especially concerning in the U.S. for some time, are now seen in emerging nations like China, Brazil, and India as well as the rest of the Western world.

Obesity is the ideal place to start because it is associated with coronary heart disease, diabetes, and some cancers. It isn't a disease per se, but rather a condition born of the malfunctioning metabolism of dietary fats thanks to the roles of blood glucose and the hormone insulin. The chart below shows how quickly obesity became prevalent in the U.S. based on data from the Center for Disease Control's NHANES surveys.

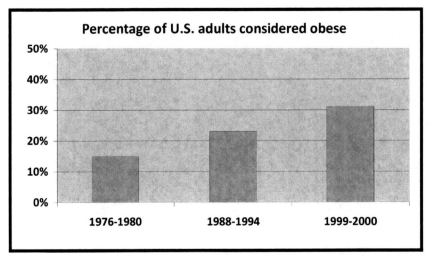

Figure 2: This bar graph shows the rise in the obesity rate of American adults between 1976 and 2000. Data is from the Center for Disease Control.

Using a BMI (Body Mass Index) cutoff of 30 kg/m², between 1976 and 1980, 15% of Americans were obese. The proportion doubled to 31% in roughly two decades.[8] Using a BMI cutoff greater than 25 kg/m², 65% of U.S. adults were overweight or obese in 2000.[9] This is 2 in every 3 American adults. Obesity may be prevalent now, but it is certainly not a new condition.

The great Indian surgeon Sushruta, considered a forefather of *Ayurveda*, observed that *medhumeda* (Sanskrit for diabetes, and literally "honey urine") developed in people with excess body fat over three millennia ago. He found that if his obese patients exercised and lost some of their body fat, they would experience fewer symptoms. Though he recorded incidences of obesity, it was exceedingly rare in ancient India.

OBESITY WAS RARE UNTIL RECENTLY

In fact, obesity was rare throughout modern human history until very recently, and American insurance records illustrate this fact. Since the 1950s, insurance companies have factored in their clients' body weight when determining premiums as they began to recognize the link between being obese and having heart attacks.[10] But the obesity rate

17

did not take off in the U.S. until the 1980s, which shows exactly when Americans began eating less dietary fats and more carbohydrates.

While obesity was always historically associated with wealth, it is more associated with poverty in modern times. This may explain why societies that are poor by Western standards are experiencing obesity epidemics. In 1997, the World Health Organization (WHO) acknowledged that obesity was a global problem after examining data from nations like Mexico, and the WHO paper asserts that obesity became widespread due to urbanization, which promotes a less active lifestyle and provides easier access to processed foods, and the industrialization of food, which had led to an oversupply of low-cost energy-dense foods.

These two processes, urbanization and industrialization of food, have been witnessed throughout history. Dr. Rob Thompson, author of "The Glycemic Load Diet," writes that 10,000 years ago, people in the Mediterranean and Indian subcontinent learned how to cultivate wheat and rice and extract their starchy seeds through the primitive process of grinding the husks between rocks. Over hundreds of generations, people in these fertile lands began making grounded wheat and rice taste better by adding fat from meat and milk products, lightening them with yeast to make breads, and eating sugar with them for sweetness.

Starvation was very common throughout man's existence, and these lightly refined carbohydrates provided nutrition and, most importantly, energy. Cultivation and light refining of whole grains made civilization possible in Mesopotamia and South Asia, and these practices spread throughout Asia, Europe, and Africa. The idea of refining these grains to make them more edible and last longer in storage also spread.

Whereas wheat and rice were the grains of the Old World, corn was the staple of New World peoples. Another plant from the Americas, the starchy tuber we call the potato, provided an abundance of calories and carbohydrates to early man and became popular in the Old World. Similar to red chili peppers, the potato was brought to

India from outside. The Spaniards brought the potato from Peru to Europe, where it spread like wildfire, and the Portuguese brought it to India.[iv]

If refined carbohydrates are linked directly to obesity today, why was obesity not prevalent in the past? There are several reasons for this. First, portions were small because food was scarcer and more expensive. The notable exceptions were people with great wealth who could afford to eat lots of milled wheat and potatoes. Portraits show that many royals and merchants were overweight, and during these periods obesity was a status symbol and considered attractive. Even during times of relative prosperity for the middle class, such as in Victorian England, people's portions were small compared with portion sizes of today, especially in the U.S. Second, people constantly walked from place to place or were engaged in hard labor. Third, most people ate grains that were not as refined as they are today.

INDUSTRIALIZATION OF FOOD

Throughout the 1800s, as the pace of industrialization accelerated, food became cheaper and more processed. Around this time, more people became wealthy enough to buy more food. By the early 1900s, people in the U.S. and U.K. were eating more food than they had ever had in the past. Around this time, the rates of people carrying excessive body fat rose but remained at less than 10% of adults in both countries. Compare that with today, where about 30% of American adults are obese and more than 60% are overweight.

Doctors noted that rates of people with too much body fat actually fell during the Great Depression, explained by a scarcity of food, but this drop was temporary. As the U.S. economy boomed following World War II, factories began focusing on making all kinds of products for the home, including food. Food became even cheaper because of these efforts, and Americans began eating more again.

[iv] *Batata* is the word for potato in Portuguese, as it is in western Indian languages where the Portuguese based their colonies.

Big companies began to heavily refine grains, thereby stripping them of their nutrition and fiber. By the 1950s, white bread, made of heavily refined wheat flour, became one of the most commonly purchased food products. Americans also started eating more red meat, butter, and sugar than ever before.

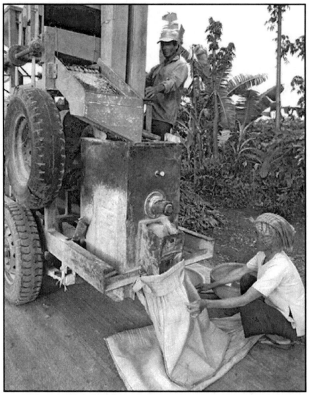

Figure 3: Rice mill on wheels. (Photo used under Creative Commons from International Rice Research Institute Images.)

DIETARY FATS BLAMED FOR HEART DISEASE

In the 1950s, physicians and researchers noted that more people were entering hospitals with coronary heart disease. In fact, some physicians had never been trained on how to treat heart attacks, as it was relatively uncommon before this time. Researchers began to scrutinize American diets to find an explanation. Their early work revealed that

Americans were eating more dietary fats than ever before. Americans were also eating more carbohydrates from refined grains, but this was lost on researchers because overall there wasn't a significant change in the average person's consumption of carbohydrates overall, as carbohydrates from refined grains replaced those from whole grains.

Dr. Ancel Keys, a University of Minnesota researcher who became the leading voice on nutrition and health in post-war America, linked dietary fat and dietary cholesterol to coronary heart disease. The saying "You are what you eat," expressing that people gained excess body fat because they were eating too much dietary fat, became dogma even in the medical community. Keys and another influential nutrition researcher named Dr. Jean Mayer at Harvard ignored the few researchers who connected the rise in heart disease to the rise in refined grains in the diet. And when the link between high cholesterol levels and heart attacks was described in the literature, doctors told people to eat fewer fats and more carbs.

Advocacy groups like the American Heart Association (AHA) and government agencies like the U.S. Department of Agriculture (USDA) bought into the "lipid hypothesis" and began telling the public that dietary fats caused obesity and heart disease. The campaigners demonized red meat, eggs, and milk and said people should replace them with carbohydrate-rich foods like products made of flour and rice as well as potatoes. Big companies making these kinds of foods saw an opportunity and immediately jumped on the bandwagon with their well-funded marketing departments. Americans of course listened.

SIMPLE CARBOHYDRATES AND THE LINK TO OBESITY AND HEART DISEASE

Dr. Thompson explains in his book on the Glycemic Load diet that the per capita consumption among Americans of milk fell by more than 50% between 1970 and 1997. On the other hand, the per capita consumption of rice increased by more than 180% within the same timeframe. He also described a close association between the rise in the per capita consumption of wheat (most of which is heavily refined) and the percentage of Americans considered obese between 1960 and 2000. The chart below illustrates those two trends.

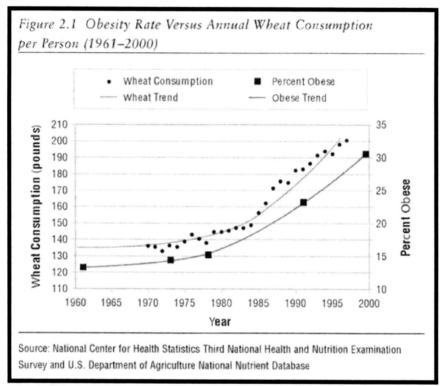

Figure 2.1 Obesity Rate Versus Annual Wheat Consumption per Person (1961–2000)

Source: National Center for Health Statistics Third National Health and Nutrition Examination Survey and U.S. Department of Agriculture National Nutrient Database

Figure 4: This graph shows the close association between the consumption of wheat per capita (light line) and the obesity rate (heavy line) in the United States between 1960 and 2000. Reprinted from "Glycemic Load Diet" by Rob Thompson, M.D.[11]

Not only were Americans eating more refined grains, such as breads, pastas, chips, cookies, and frozen meals, they were drinking more sugary sodas. Simply put, the decades when obesity rose and became an epidemic in the U.S. were the same decades where the average American ate more simple, easy-to-digest carbohydrates, as in more wheat, rice, potatoes, corn and corn products like high fructose corn syrup, and sucrose or table sugar, and less dietary fats, as in milk, dairy products, and some meats. During this period, the death rate from heart attacks went down, but the rate of people developing coronary heart disease did not fall.

You may correctly conclude, as several health experts have, that the rises in obesity and coronary heart disease were due to people eating more easily digestible carbs from *refined* grains (whose consumption rose), and not from fatty foods (whose consumption actually fell). This story explains what is happening around the world. Globalization has made more people relatively wealthier, especially in emerging nations like India, China, and Brazil.

With greater wealth, people buy more food. This has attracted companies that manufacture food products, including those companies that make products from refined grains like white rice and finely ground wheat flour, thus making more processed and refined food available. As their marketing techniques get people hooked, and people move away from where foods in their more natural state are easily accessible, people are increasingly eating more refined grains.

Let me say right here that easier access to food is of course a good thing, but the evidence points to easier access to energy-rich, nutrition-poor foods being behind the epidemics of obesity, heart disease, and diabetes all over the world. In an ideal world, access to *whole* and *natural* foods like fresh vegetables and fruits, legumes and nuts, spices and herbs would be improved. In addition, companies would sell grains that are lightly refined such as brown rice and coarse, stone-milled wholemeal, as they are more nutrient-dense.

However, in the real world, the increasing presence of refined carbs, starchy foods, and sugars in the modern diets explains the dramatic rise in chronic disease. Recall that our ancestors ate *whole, natural* foods over tens of thousands of years. Thus, the human body evolved to handle these foods efficiently. *Unnatural, processed* foods are new in the history of man, and thus the human body is not capable of handling large amounts of simple carbohydrates well or functioning normally without vital minerals, vitamins, and antioxidants. The human body becomes stressed when the input is poor, so to speak. The glucose-insulin feedback system begins to malfunction, and the body's immune system cannot control inflammation as well.

23

Understanding Chronic Disease

It is health that is real wealth and not pieces of gold and silver.

– Mahatma Gandhi

The past several generations have seen a rise in chronic disease. Some of this is explained by the fact that people are living longer. In the past, many died of infections, malnutrition, or violence before reaching middle age, where chronic diseases usually begin to emerge. But the explosive rise in heart disease, diabetes, and some cancers as well as obesity in the last two generations cannot be explained by longevity alone. As I illustrated earlier, the significant rise has in large part been due to increasing consumption of processed foods containing refined grains, sugars, and starches. This is the "carbohydrate hypothesis."

In my opinion, it should be called the "simple, easily-digested carbohydrate hypothesis." After all, the British Indian physician Robert McCarrison blamed white rice, flour, and sugar for certain groups in India having high rates of illness, not vegetables or legumes, which are also carbohydrate-dense. Regardless of the name, this makes sense when you understand how glucose, a sugar molecule digested into the bloodstream from carbohydrates, interacts with insulin, and the role excess body fat plays in inflammation.

The carbohydrate hypothesis is no longer controversial. Thanks to insights by the likes of Mr. Gary Taubes, who wrote "Good Calories, Bad Calories," and advocacy by people like Dr. Walter Willett of Harvard, America's pre-eminent nutritionist-physician, the word is getting out. What I explain in this book is *not* new, as McCarrison's words from the 1930s reveal. But you as the reader will get much benefit from better understanding what evidence from the forgotten past and recent scientific studies tell us.

To help affix those strands of information firmly on your own knowledge tree, or if you want to dive deeper into the science, read the upcoming section on chronic diseases and the basics of food. However, if all you want is to learn what constitutes a healthy Indian diet and recipes that fit this profile, skip this section altogether.

I will keep it as simple and concise as possible. Actually, much of what I write will be easy to follow because you will have come across certain concepts before. You may have a relative living with chronic disease, making you familiar with some of the terms I use. The new paradigms on the glucose-insulin feedback system and the role of inflammation may be more technical, but they are not difficult to follow. I have documented the claims in this section in the Endnotes of the book should you wish to read the source material.

CORONARY HEART DISEASE

Atherosclerosis and Plaques

When doctors tell people they have heart disease, they usually mean atherosclerosis, also called coronary heart disease. Atherosclerosis is characterized by the formation of plaques inside the walls of coronary arteries, which supply the heart with fresh blood. The plaques can narrow the space inside the affected arteries through which blood flows. If the space becomes too narrow, the amounts of oxygen and nutrients that get to the corresponding heart muscle become less than normal. Eventually this causes chest pain, which doctors call angina and see as the first sign of clinically significant heart disease.

The plaques are made of yellow fatty material produced by the unsuccessful ingestion by macrophages, a white blood cell, of low-density lipoproteins containing cholesterol (LDL-C). While flowing freely in the blood, an LDL-C may injure the inner wall of a coronary artery. This same particle may then lodge into the wall or allow other lipoproteins downstream to enter the site of the injury.

25

Free radicals in the site of injury, created as an initial inflammatory response to the injury by white blood cells, oxidize the LDL particles. Oxidized LDL particles, when ingested, trigger an inflammatory response attracting more white blood cells, and oxidized LDL particles cannot be normally processed. Thus, macrophages that ingest these cholesterol-containing particles rupture.

Partially digested cholesterol, lipoprotein, and white cell matter build up inside the atherosclerotic plaques, triggering more inflammation. They grow larger, and the inflamed arterial wall becomes stiffer, which causes the narrowing of the arterial space. As you can see, inflammation plays a prominent role in the formation of coronary atherosclerotic plaques.

Some researchers believe an immune system that lets inflammation continue unabated promotes atherosclerosis, and they cite a body of evidence that shows certain infections (known to elevate the general level of inflammation) are associated with increased incidences of coronary disease.[12] While association does not prove cause, the new medical consensus based on this and other evidence is that there is a connection between LDL-C particles, inflammation, and coronary heart disease.

Inflammation and Heart Attacks

The untreated growth of atherosclerotic plaques, driven largely by inflammation and small, dense LDL particles (rather than large LDL particles) will usually lead to chest pain. A heart attack is caused when an arterial plaque ruptures. The inflamed yellow, fatty material inside the plaque is exposed to fresh blood flowing through the coronary artery, which triggers a different type of inflammatory response, one using coagulation factors and platelets. A large clot (or thrombus) quickly forms.

The clot blocks blood flow more effectively than plaques. The catastrophic event called a heart attack (or myocardial infarction) happens when the clot grows to fill the entire arterial space or breaks free and blocks a smaller arterial space downstream. The obstruction may be temporary, but it is bad enough to cause severe injury to the heart muscle. When the obstruction is more permanent, some heart muscle can die.

What causes a plaque to rupture in the first place? Inflammation, the kind where white blood cells eat into the thin endothelial tissue left between the plaque and fresh blood in the arterial space. Another kind of inflammation forms the clot at the plaque site. Incidentally, the death of heart muscle from a heart attack doesn't kill; a resulting heart arrhythmia (or abnormal heart rhythm) usually does.

Treating Heart Disease

Coronary heart disease is treated in many ways. Early on, patients are started on medication like aspirin, which is essentially an anti-inflammatory. They are counseled to stop smoking, improve their diets, and get more exercise. Diseases that increase the risk of heart attack, primarily diabetes and arrhythmias, are medically treated. Patients are often started on statins, which not only lower cholesterol but also inflammation.

If significant symptoms like chest pain are experienced, patients are given medicine called beta blockers, calcium channel blockers, and nitroglycerides. At this point, a cardiologist may do a coronary angiography (or "heart cath") to see how narrowed the arteries have become. He may even open an obstructed coronary artery and insert a stent to keep it open. If the narrowing is severe and widespread, a surgeon may perform coronary arterial bypass graft surgery (also called CABG or simply "bypass surgery"). The consequences of severe coronary disease and heart attacks, such as heart failure, are managed with medicine and devices like Intermittent Cardiac Defibrillators (ICDs).

Interestingly, newer research shows lifestyle changes, including adopting a plant-based diet, can help people better manage their coronary disease. In the late 1990s, the cardiologist Dr. Ornish showed that people could stop or even reverse atherosclerosis with an intensive lifestyle regimen ("10% fat whole foods vegetarian diet, aerobic exercise, stress-management training, smoking cessation, group psychosocial support"), which was unheard of before.[13] Plaque-filled arteries actually opened up in patients who kept with Ornish's program. These patients had fewer heart attacks than the control patients in the study, who were treated conventionally and made some changes, and whose arteries continued to narrow.

Saturated Fats and Heart Disease

In the sphere of public health, health groups have campaigned to have people lower their LDL-C levels by changing their diets. The USDA, AHA, and American Diabetes Association have advocated a low-fat, low-cholesterol diet with the idea that if people eat less of them, they will lower their blood cholesterol levels.[14]

However, telling people to reduce their dietary fats is the wrong approach according to nutrition experts like Dr. Walter Willett at Harvard. He has counseled people to have more monounsaturated fats, like those in olive oil, as they reduce a person's risk of developing coronary heart disease. The call to reduce all fats has meant that people have also cut beneficial fats out of their diets.

Furthermore, the science isn't clear on whether all saturated fats are bad. Just as it was useful earlier to differentiate between refined grains and whole grains, we must differentiate long-chain saturated fats from short and medium-chain saturated fats because only long-chain saturated fats seem to have a detrimental effect on cholesterol levels.

A meta-analysis of 60 trials showed that a diet high in lauric acid, a medium-chain saturated fat that is abundant in coconut oil, was associated with an increase in the HDL-C to LDL-C ratio (that is, good to bad cholesterol). Lauric acid improved cholesterol levels in this way more substantially than any fat – saturated or unsaturated.[15] Thus, not all saturated fats are bad in terms of heart health.

While the science is unclear on saturated fats because of the clumsy way earlier research grouped them together, science is clear on trans fats. These are bad, as trans fats increase a person's risk of developing coronary disease and heart attacks more than any other molecule found in food.

A WORD ON STROKES

Basically a "brain attack," in most cases strokes are caused when a clot forms and blocks off an artery supplying fresh blood to a part of the brain. Clots causing strokes usually form elsewhere in the body. Stress, like high blood pressure or a heart arrhythmia, causes the clot to travel into the brain. When oxygen and nutrients can't get to brain tissue because of the clot, the tissue experiences a severe injury or death. Some strokes don't cause permanent or significant injury to the patient, but some do and can leave people handicapped or dead.

Risk factors for strokes are the same as for heart attacks: smoking, diabetes, bad cholesterol levels, and high blood pressure.[v] It is better to prevent rather than treat strokes, so doctors start patients at risk on aspirin, which reduces the risk of the kind of inflammation that causes clotting. They also treat diseases like atrial fibrillation, hypertension and diabetes.

DIABETES AND INSULIN RESISTANCE

"Sugar Disease"

You may think of diabetes as "sugar disease," and rightly so. Indeed, the disease is diagnosed and managed by testing one's blood glucose – the most common form of sugar in the blood. The consequences of poorly treated diabetes, namely diseases of the nerves, eyes, heart, kidneys, and arteries, are caused by high blood sugar. But diabetes is actually a disease of the glucose-insulin feedback system, which controls fat metabolism in the body, among other processes.

The hormone insulin is made by the pancreas in response to higher than normal blood glucose levels (like after eating food) and tells muscle, liver, and fat cells to take glucose out of the blood and use it or store it as glycogen (in the liver) and triglycerides (in fat and muscle cells) for future use.

---

[v] Atrial fibrillation is an exception and one of the most important risk factors for strokes.

Normally, the glucose (and other sugars like fructose) that enters the blood will be used for energy or stored, depending on the insulin level. When insulin is high, glucose is stored. When glucose levels normalize thanks to the insulin signal, the pancreas stops releasing insulin. When insulin becomes low or normal, this tells cells in the body to use glucose now for energy and to not store it as triglycerides (essentially molecular fat) or glycogen.

Glucose-Insulin Feedback System and Insulin Resistance

This feedback system between insulin and glucose goes wrong in diabetes. Either insulin is not being produced by the pancreas, as in type 1 diabetes mellitus, which usually starts early in life and is treated by self-injected insulin. But type 1 is rare compared with type 2, which makes up 80% of diabetes cases. In type 2 diabetes mellitus, insulin is made, but its signaling power is weak. Muscle, liver, and fat cells basically ignore what the insulin is telling them.

This is a simple illustration of "insulin resistance." Type 2 diabetes is associated with obesity, heart disease, and metabolic syndrome. However, a person can have insulin resistance, a bad health condition itself, but not develop full-blown diabetes until much later in life.

The causes of insulin resistance are multi-factorial, but two processes stand out: chronically elevated levels of insulin and obesity. Recall that insulin levels become high when glucose levels become high, after a meal for example. If the meal contains a lot of carbohydrates, this translates to even higher blood glucose levels after the carbs are digested, and then even higher levels of insulin. If all or at least most of a person's meals are high in carbohydrates, insulin levels will be chronically elevated. The condition of chronically high insulin levels encourages cells to stop listening so intently to what the insulin has to say. In other words, cells will begin ignoring insulin.

Excess body fat (or obesity in other words) promotes the development of insulin resistance because fat tissue releases cytokines, which are inflammatory molecules that tell the body's cells to use less glucose. This is to allow immune cells involved in inflammation to have more glucose for energy. The supposed link between all these conditions and diseases is that obesity promotes insulin resistance (and both obesity and insulin are promoted by high amounts of carbohydrates in the diet), which in turn promotes the development of diabetes.

Treating Diabetes

The first thing doctors do in a newly-diagnosed diabetic patient is advise them to change their diet and to exercise. Unfortunately, patients are not always given clear instructions on what kind of changes to make, and they are often challenged to make those changes because of old habits. Sometimes doctors will prescribe medications that help the body's cells respond properly to the insulin signal. The first medication is usually metformin. If the patient's blood glucose levels over time remain high (based on her hemoglobin A1c), then other oral anti-diabetic medications such as sulfonylureas and thiazolidinediones are prescribed.

Chronic insulin resistance, as experienced by long-term type 2 diabetics, strains the pancreas. Insulin production thus begins to slow down, and type 2 diabetics eventually have the same basic problem as type 1 diabetics, which is that the pancreas stops producing insulin. At this point, an endocrinologist will manage the disease with self-injected insulin and continue with oral anti-diabetic medications, as type 2 diabetes is essentially a disease of insulin resistance (or where cells ignore insulin). The long-term consequences of poorly controlled diabetes are kidney failure, blindness, heart attacks, strokes, and potentially some cancers thanks in large part to the actions of excess body fat.

Newer techniques show that changes to diet can help people better manage their advanced diabetes. While the ADA advocates a low-fat diet with up to 130 grams of carbs every day, Dr. Richard K. Berstein, who helped start the self-monitoring of glucose patient movement in the 1980s, advocates a very low carb diet of no more than 30 grams a day for optimal blood glucose control.

Even a moderate amount of daily carbohydrates helped people with diabetes improve their blood glucose and insulin levels as well as risk factors for heart disease in several studies.[16] In a study of ten type 2 diabetic, obese patients, a very low-carbohydrate diet forced physicians to decrease insulin doses in two people and thiazolidinedione and metformin doses in one, and stop sulfonylureas altogether in a fourth patient.[17] These are telltale signs that what one eats daily can not only prevent diabetes, but it can also successfully treat it.

OBESITY AND BELLY FAT

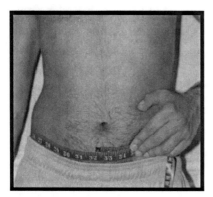

Figure 5: The AHA, in its endorsement of criteria for diagnosing metabolic syndrome, states a waist circumference of 40 inches (102 cm) and more for men, and 35 inches (88 cm) and more for women, represents having too much central body fat.i

Obesity (specifically central obesity, which is also called abdominal fat, belly fat, or beer belly) is a medical condition – not a disease per se – where the accumulation of excess body fat is so great that it harms your health. Professionals use two methods to determine whether a person is obese. The more popular method is by calculating the patient's Body Mass Index. A BMI greater than 30 kg/m^2 defines obesity, while a BMI greater than 25 kg/m^2 defines being overweight. The other method is by measuring one's waist circumference (not the hips, see the picture above). The AHA, in its endorsement of criteria for diagnosing metabolic syndrome, states a waist circumference of 40 inches (102 cm) and more for men, and 35 inches (88 cm) and more for women, represents having too much central body fat.[18]

The kind of fat cells (or adipocytes) that leads to clinically significant obesity is different from other kinds of fat cells. Obesity (i.e., excess abdominal or central fat) is a condition of excess *visceral* fat cells, which become yellow and greasy tissues that sit over the intestines in our abdominal cavity. In contrast, subcutaneous fat is underneath the skin, and intermuscular fat is between muscle fibers, and they don't contribute to obesity or its associated diseases.

According to both evidence and the logic of the carbohydrate hypothesis, visceral fat grows when insulin levels are chronically high – due to insulin resistance.[19,20] This in turn causes visceral fat cells to use more glucose (and fatty acids) from the blood and create more triglycerides, a form of molecular fat that is ideal for storage inside cells. As visceral fat tissues grow, they behave like an endocrine organ, meaning they secrete hormones and inflammatory molecules called adipokines to act on different parts of the body. The idea is that adipokines help visceral fat tissue grow by making the body's other cells insulin resistant. If these cells don't use glucose, more is left in the blood for the growing visceral fat cells to use, again for energy and growth. In this way, visceral fat tissue behaves similar to a cancerous tumor, which also releases chemicals into the blood to help itself grow at the expense of the rest of the body.

Central obesity is dangerous. This is because its mere presence is associated with a statistically higher risk of coronary heart disease, diabetes, high blood pressure, bad cholesterol levels, and insulin resistance.[21] Therefore, central to preventing these diseases and conditions is the prevention of obesity.

Modern diets, being based largely on simple, easily digestible carbohydrates from refined grains, sugars, and starchy plants like potatoes, encourage the development of obesity. Changing your diet to make it less based on these "bad carbs" will pay dividends. The healthy Indian diet, which is based on good carbohydrates found in leafy green plants and fruit, which also come with fiber, protein in legumes, and dietary fats in dairies, are low on these "bad carbs."

METABOLIC SYNDROME

Some physicians began grouping together risk factors for both diabetes and coronary disease under the umbrella term "metabolic syndrome" in the 1950s. The term then fell out of fashion as

33

specialists focused on each disease separately. But research continued, and in 1988, Stanford endocrinologist Dr. Gerald Reaven gave an ADA lecture summarizing the links between insulin resistance and both coronary disease and diabetes, thereby bringing the concept back en vogue.

Today, metabolic syndrome describes a condition, not a disease, based on five criteria:

- Central obesity (e.g., abdominal fat, belly fat, or beer belly)

- High blood pressure

- Insulin resistance/high blood sugar

- High triglycerides

- Low HDL-cholesterol

Because the condition is still not well defined (i.e., each health advocacy group has its own specific criteria with some overlap), there is no consensus on how to treat it.[22]

Your takeaway from learning about metabolic syndrome is to understand that coronary heart disease and diabetes are both promoted by insulin resistance. Insulin resistance develops when the glucose/insulin feedback system stops working normally. This happens in large part due to the regular consumption of too many simple carbohydrates that are found in refined grains, starches, and sugars, which stress the body with large surges of glucose and insulin.

Also, insulin resistance is promoted by obesity (i.e., excess visceral fat tissue), which creates an environment making the body even more insulin resistant. Visceral fat uses more glucose for both energy and to create triglycerides for storage.[vi] Triglycerides and its derivative molecular fats are released into the blood, compounding the harmful effects of high blood glucose, which is a direct consequence of cells becoming resistant to insulin.

[vi] The liver also uses free fatty acids released by visceral fat tissue to make and release triglycerides.

The goal then, to prevent or manage metabolic syndrome (whether or not you have heart disease and diabetes), is to avoid becoming insulin resistant and gaining excessive body fat. You have the power to control this to some extent by keeping the amounts of bad carbs, that is carbohydrates from processed foods and starchy plants like potatoes, low in what you eat.

CANCERS

Cancer is not One Disease but Many Similar Diseases

Few words strike fear into people's hearts like the word "cancer." Being diagnosed with cancer used to be, and still is in many cases, considered a death sentence, though rates of survival and even cure for some cancers have improved over the last several decades. It is important to understand that there is not one single cancer that affects multiple parts of the body; rather, each organ can have its own kind of cancer. Within each organ, each type of cell can have its own cancer, and the risk factors for each different cancer are themselves different. As an illustration, the hormone estrogen increases one's risk of ovarian cancer, but not of thyroid cancer.

Likewise, inflammation of the thyroid gland may lead to one kind of thyroid cancer (papillary) but not another (medullary thyroid cancer). Yet, some carcinogens increase the risk of many cancers, and tobacco is the best example of this. Something must connect these cancers together if risk factors are similar. Certain principles tie all cancers together. All cancer cells, no matter the type, are characterized by uncontrolled growth.

All cancers tend to invade adjacent tissues, and all cancers seek to metastasize to distant parts of the body. In general, cancers are triggered by random mutations or changes in a cell's DNA, and are then driven by hormonal changes (e.g., obesity increases the incidence of breast cancers because excess fat cells drive up the level of estrogen) and inflammation (e.g., in some people the bacteria *Helicobacter pylori* induces inflammation in the stomach, creating an environment ripe for gastric cancer to grow.

35

ENVIRONMENT TRUMPS GENETICS IN CANCER DEVELOPMENT

More people are developing cancers than in the past because people are living longer, but experts believe that the rise cannot be explained by this fact alone. They blame physical, chemical, and biological carcinogens common in our environments. Chemicals that people lived with, such as asbestos and amaranth dye, were banned because they induced cancers. Bisphenol A (BPA) may promote cancer growth by acting as a hormone – according to a 2010 review – and surely other chemicals in our environment will be linked to cancers in the future.[23]

Despite evidence to the contrary, people believe a person develops cancer largely because his genes are defective. But this isn't true. Rarely will the DNA you were born with, the same DNA in each cell of your body, cause or promote cancer. In fact, your genes were designed to prevent cancer or destroy cancer cells early. There is a connection, however. When the DNA molecule is injured by random mutation, inflammation, or carcinogen in a particular cell, the injury may turn off a tumor suppression gene or turn on an oncogene. While mutations occur randomly with little to no outside influence, inflammation is triggered by environmental causes.

And carcinogens are a part of the environment. Researchers estimated that 90-95% of cases of cancers are caused by "environmental factors" that turn genes on and off. Their work showed that nearly one in every 3 cancers was caused by tobacco, one by a poor diet and obesity, and one by factors we have less control over like exposure to UV rays and ionizing radiation.[24] The World Healthy Organization (WHO) estimated that one in every 3 cancers is completely preventable if they avoid tobacco, obesity, a low intake of fruits and vegetables, physical *in*activity, alcohol, sexually transmitted infections, and air pollution.[25]

Treating Cancers

Each cancer is unique, so it is impossible to fully explain here how they are treated, but generally, if the cancer is just one tumor accessible to a surgeon, it will be taken out. If a tumor cannot be taken out safely, targeted radiation therapy or chemotherapy is used. Unfortunately, most cancers are discovered by patients and doctors when they have already invaded healthy tissues and even metastasized to distant organs.

After a battery of lab and imaging studies map out what kind of cancer it is, where it is, and how far it has traveled, the oncologist will begin chemotherapy in most cases and consult with a surgeon and radiation oncologist if other kinds of therapy are needed. Cancers tend to be tricky, and some can resist conventional therapies. Thus, new experimental agents that are not yet proven to work are sometimes used against a cancer.

Unlike coronary heart disease or diabetes, doctors do not always tell their cancer patients to improve their diets. However, landmark research on turmeric by Dr. Bharat Aggarwal at M.D. Anderson Cancer Center in Houston should change people's perspective on using food as medicine. As should the work of Dr. Ornish at the University of California, San Francisco, whose team have demonstrated that intensive lifestyle changes can mildly slow the progression of early, low-grade prostate cancer, unlike conventional therapies using surgery, radiation, and anti-testosterone medications, which do not slow the progression.[26]

Here are the lifestyle changes in that study.

> [An] intensive lifestyle program that included a vegan diet supplemented with soy (1 daily serving of tofu plus 58 gm of a fortified soy protein powdered beverage), fish oil (3 gm daily), vitamin E (400 IU daily), selenium (200 mcg daily) and vitamin C (2 gm daily), moderate aerobic exercise (walking 30 minutes 6 days weekly), stress management techniques (gentle yoga based stretching, breathing, meditation, imagery and progressive relaxation for a total of 60 minutes daily) and participation in a 1-hour support group once weekly to enhance adherence to the intervention.

This lifestyle regimen is difficult for most people to follow. But the study is insightful because it shows how an exclusively plant-based diet supplemented by vitamins and exercise, yoga, and meditation can help the body fight cancer.

NEW PARADIGM #1: INFLAMMATION AND CHRONIC DISEASES

How Inflammation Normally Works

When a part of your body gets injured, cells of nearby blood vessels signal platelets in the blood to arrive at the site. A system of other molecules called coagulation factors is triggered, and your blood get "stickier" to form a clot to stop bleeding at the site. Platelets then signal white blood cells to arrive. In the injury site, macrophages, B cells, and T cells, release molecules called cytokines. They include prostaglandins, thromboxanes, leukotrienes, and chemokines like TGF-α.

These molecules help your body's white blood cells coordinate both an attack against offending agents like bacteria and a quick-fix repair operation. The cytokines also tell blood vessels to let more immune cells into the local area. After some time, the acute phases of attacking and quick-fix repairing are over, and other white blood cells signal fibroblasts to create a scar. After some more time, the local inflammatory response will shut down and normal cells may re-grow in or around the injury site.

Usually, the previously injured tissue will be restored as much as possible to normal function. This is generally true whether the injury is a bacteria pneumonia or viral cold, a visible stab wound in the abdomen or a microscopic tear in an artery from the physical stress of high blood pressure. Inflammatory processes like the one I have described happen constantly. When the immune system is well regulated, it orchestrates various cells and molecules to behave effectively, works in harmony with the tissue when the injury has occurred, and finally brings the entire operation to a close. In this context, inflammation benefits us greatly. It is when the immune system stops working like it should and inflammation occurs without proper regulation that disease can form or grow.

Inflammation and Cancers

In his book "Anticancer," Dr. Servan-Schreiber wrote that more than 100 years ago the German physician Dr. Rudolph Virchow noticed that cancer tended to develop in many patients at the exact spot where they had previously received a traumatic injury. Under the microscope, these tumors contained an abundance of white blood cells, the kind involved in inflammation. In 1986, Dr. Harold Dvorak at Harvard Medical School published an essay in the *New England Journal of Medicine* describing the similarity between processes that govern stromal cancer formation and wound healing, thereby linking cancer to inflammation.[27]

Dr. Dvorak pointed out that one cancer in six is directly linked to a chronic inflammatory state. For example, cervical cancer is strongly associated with the HPV virus, stomach cancer with *H. pylori*, liver cancer with the chronic hepatitis B or C viruses, mesothelioma with inflammation caused by the presence of asbestos, non-small cell lung cancer with inflammation triggered by the invasion of the many toxic chemicals in processed tobacco, and colon cancer with chronic inflammatory bowel disease.

More research supported the new paradigm linking cancer to inflammation, and it received serious thought leading up to the 2005 meeting hosted by the U.S. National Cancer Institute to discuss the role inflammation plays in the formation and growth of cancer.[28] The NCI report explained how cancers manage to trick the body's immune system, designed to attack and heal, into helping tumors grow at the expense of the body.

To sustain their growth, cancer cells release the same molecular signals immune cells do to get resources like glucose and amino acids (the basic building blocks of cells) from the body. Cancer cells use these substances to also invade surrounding tissues. Unlike your body's normal immune system, cancer cells don't stop releasing these pro-inflammatory molecules. One consequence is that cancer cells don't die from apoptosis (or self-death, which most of your cells are programmed to do), so they keep growing.

Your immune system is capable of killing cancer cells. A specific white blood cell called the "Natural Killer cell" (NK cell) attacks cancer cells and prevents them from growing into tumors that are too large and active for the immune system to handle, but when a tumor grows that big, it is able to hijack the immune system and thus escape detection, preventing other white blood cells from attacking.[29]

Another body of evidence supporting the hypothesis that connects cancer to abnormal inflammation is made of studies showing that people who regularly take anti-inflammatory drugs are less likely to develop cancers over the long term.[30] A recent meta-analysis of about 25,000 people demonstrated that people taking a daily aspirin, a non-steroidal anti-inflammatory drug (NSAID) that decreases prostaglandin and thromboxane production, died less of several common cancers compared with people who didn't take a daily aspirin.[31]

A Central Inflammatory Player in Cancers

Based on recent science, the inflammatory molecule pathways being most squarely blamed is regulated by NF-kappa B. This protein is one of several that controls the process of converting DNA into mRNA, which is then translated into other proteins. NF-kappa B specifically promotes the production of proteins that help cells live longer and avoid pre-programmed self-death (i.e., apoptosis). What activates NF-kappa B? Stresses, from pro-inflammatory cytokines to free radicals, UV radiation, oxidized LDL particles, and bacterial or viral antigens.[32] An injury to the cell often damages its DNA so badly that the cell dies.

However, if NF-kappa B is somehow activated, which often happens, the cell survives by stopping the process of self-death. NF-kappa B also helps the cell produce signals to white blood cells to create local inflammation in the hopes of ridding the stressor, whether it be a toxin, free radical, or bacteria. Cancers always rig the system: They keep NF-kappa B activated and thus avoid self-death, and also grow into a tumor.

If you can see cancers under this new paradigm, that is as inflammatory diseases or simply encouraged by inflammation to grow, you can see why some oncology researchers view NF-kappa B as the holy grail of treatment.[33] Companies are already spending millions on developing medications to target NF-kappa B and another molecule I described earlier, TNF-alpha (which triggers the NF-kappa B pathway) or molecules triggered downstream by NF-kappa B.

While companies are devoting a lot of time, effort, and money, a bioactive molecule in a natural spice in Indian cooking is already close to that holy grail. It reduces the activation of NF-kappa B and reduces the growth of some cancerous human cells studied in an MD Anderson Cancer Center laboratory. That component is curcumin, which is found in turmeric powder, itself an essential part of curry powders and *garam masala* (mix of hot spices).[34]

Inflammation and Obesity, Heart Disease, and Diabetes

Excess visceral fat tissue behaves like an endocrine organ, producing signal molecules called adipokines. IL-6 promotes widespread inflammation, for example. Other adipokines promote platelet activation and make the blood stickier, thereby promoting clot formation, and TNF-alpha encourages cancer cells to grow (by amplifying NF-kappa B). TNF-alpha from visceral fat also promotes insulin resistance, which also leads to diabetes and heart disease but is believed to play a pro-cancer role.[35]

That excess visceral fat encourages inflammation may explain why obesity is linked to many cancers. The National Cancer Institute lists breast, endometrial, colon, esophageal, and kidney cancers as strongly associated with excess body fat.[36] It has been observed in the same literature that getting rid of some visceral fat reduces the risk of developing some of these cancers (just as doing so reduces the risk of developing heart disease and diabetes). This benefit from reducing the amount of visceral fat probably has something to do with there being less adipokines like IL-6 and TNF-alpha, which promote inflammation.

Evidence also links inflammation to heart disease. Recall that inflammation is triggered after a coronary artery is injured. This is followed by the invasion of immune cells, which create an endless cycle of local inflammation, as they are incapable of destroying oxidized LDL-cholesterol particles. Thus, inflammation plays a central role in the formation of atherosclerosis. Excess visceral fat tissue plays a role too, increasing the general level of inflammation and triglycerides levels, both of which are associated with a higher risk of coronary disease.[37]

Finally, evidence links inflammation to diabetes through the actions of excess visceral fat. Doctors view most type 2 diabetes cases as intimately linked, if not in fact caused by, obesity. TNF-alpha from visceral fat (i.e., obesity-related fat) promotes insulin resistance, which often leads to diabetes.[38] And it seems that a diet that promotes obesity (a diet high in easily digestible carbohydrates) itself increases inflammation. A 2008 study suggested this when overweight or obese people began eating a low-carb diet and demonstrated reduced levels of inflammatory markers like TNF-alpha and IL-6 in the blood.[39]

NEW PARADIGM #2: BAD CARBS, INSULIN RESISTANCE, AND CHRONIC DISEASES

Rise in Sugar and Refined Grains Linked to Rise in Diabetes Historically

In 1907, Dr. Havelock Charles, president of the Medical Board of India, hosted a symposium on diabetes, which he said was becoming an epidemic among the "lazy and indolent rich."[40] His colleague, Dr. Rai Koilas Chunder Bose of the University of Calcutta, explained that with "the progress of civilization, of higher education, and increased wealth and prosperity of the people under the British rule, the number of diabetic cases has enormously increased." What was behind this rise in diabetes in turn-of-the-century British India?

Dr. Charles believed "rice, flour, pulses and sugars," which were well loved by the "Bengali gentlemen," among whom 10% had diabetes, was responsible. (Ten percent was a high rate at the time and mirrors the 11% rate among U.S. adults in 2007).[41] Twenty years later, Dr. McCarrison noted that many Indians were eating more refined grains (milled or white rice and flour) and less traditional staples like wild rice and coarse grains (like millet and *atta* from wheat).

42

These same trends were playing out thousands of miles away among mostly white Britons. Dr. Peter Cleave, a Royal Navy physician who wrote "The Saccharine Disease," drew a chart showing the consumption of sugar per capita against the number of deaths due to diabetes in England and Wales between 1905 and 1950. What he found was a direct association between the trends, both of which had been going up except during the two world wars and the Great Depression.

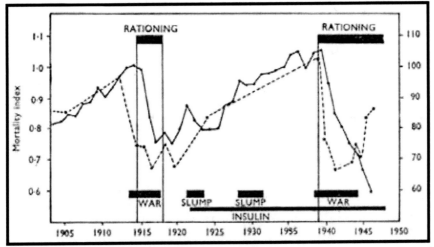

Figure 6: This graph shows the close association between the consumption of sugar per capita (dotted line) and number of deaths from diabetes (solid line) in England and Wales between 1905 and 1950. Reprinted from "The Saccharine Disease" by T.L. Cleave.[42]

Obesity Trends Up Too

During the periods where sugar and refined grain consumption went up along with the incidence of diabetes, the obesity rate also started to go up. Picking up where Dr. Cleave's chart using U.K. data left off, only one U.S. adult in ten was obese in the 1950s. Today, 3 to 4 U.S. adults out of ten are obese. Out of those same ten adults, another 3 to 4 are overweight but not obese. Note that this and other evidence demonstrates clearly that these three trends – of easily digestible carbohydrate consumption per capita, diabetes incidence, and obesity incidence – have all generally been going up since the beginning of the

20th century. Obesity has been explained as a problem of overeating. The trends suggest obesity could be better explained as an effect of overeating of refined grains, sugars, and other sources of easily digested carbs.

Moving on, obesity has also been, historically speaking, linked to wealth. It is easy to see why: A larger proportion of wealthy people were overweight compared with poor people, as hinted to in portraits since antiquity. Further evidence is that the current obesity epidemic began in the U.S. and Europe beginning around the 1970s, which were the wealthiest societies during that period, and this has since spread to wealthier parts of Asia, Africa, and the Americas.

But it would be wrong to conclude that obesity is solely related to wealth. Today's evidence shows that obesity within a society is actually more common among the poor. The journalist Gary Taubes illustrates how the hunter-gatherer Pima Indians of Arizona, once wealthy and healthy by early 1800s standards, became poor and obese by the 1850s after the U.S. government put them on reservations and gave them food rations, which the Pima spent mostly on sugar and flour. Clearly, increasing wealth did not lead to increasing fat in this society.

Obesity and Cheap Foods

And so, the association of obesity to poverty has been increasingly demonstrated around the world in recent years. This was most vividly encapsulated by an anecdote from Dr. Benjamin Caballero in the *New England Journal of Medicine*. He described seeing poor women living in the Brazilian city of São Paulo come to clinic with their children.[43] The children, thin and stunted in height for their age, were malnourished. Their mothers, on the other hand, were fat. He said it was difficult to believe the women were overeating food while letting their children starve. Rather, the insight was that both child and mother were malnourished, and that the obesity was caused by having little nutrition.

In his book "Good Calories, Bad Calories," Mr. Taubes says that general overeating, or eating more calories than a person can burn, as a cause of obesity isn't well supported by the science. There is more evidence for the hypothesis that obesity is caused by eating mostly easily digested carbohydrates, which are poor in nutrition as the refining of grains removes the fiber-rich bran and the germ where minerals and vitamins are. And why is it that the poor are more likely to become obese? Because these processed foods are actually cheaper to make and to buy than whole grain, as well as milk, meats, fruits, and vegetables.

What happened to young mothers of starving children in the slums of São Paulo also happened to the Pima Indians more than a 100 years ago: They began to eat the cheapest food available because they were poor, which happened to be flour and sugar, and then they gained excess body fat.

Other Explanations for Becoming Obese

The carbohydrate hypothesis is not the only explanation for rising obesity trends. Dr. Oz said in a brief talk that he believes chronic stress leads to the accumulation of belly fat.[44] Early humans experienced chronic stress during famines, which could last weeks to months. The body evolved to secrete hormones to compel man to find food (e.g., cannabinoids) and store fat (e.g., cortisol and insulin) for future energy use when food was scarce, which was most days. The psychological stress that modern man experiences today triggers the same hormones. But now food is readily available, especially carbohydrate-rich foods, and people become fatter.

The "lipophilia hypothesis" explains that some people are genetically programmed to become fat and others are not.[45] This is similar to how some are genetically programmed to become hairy, tall, or blonde. Now, if someone's genes express molecules that drive that person to overeat, then in this modern environment laden with carbohydrate-rich foods, it is no wonder such a person may become fat. Regardless of whether the underlying reason for how we eat is heavily influenced by our genes, we do have an enormous amount of control over how and what we eat.

Observations have shown that as Americans ate less dietary fats (less milk and *ghee*, for example), they did not become leaner. In fact, they became fatter overall during that period. Studies have shown that focusing on calories in the diet is probably misguided. A review of the Cochrane Database (considered the largest unbiased source of clinical information) demonstrated that lowering the amount of fats or calories a person eats has not translated into significant weight loss.[46] On the other hand, similar studies have shown that a low-carb diet (like the Atkins ketogenic diet) is better than low-fat and low-calorie diets in two ways: at causing weight loss and helping the person maintain weight loss.[47]

Insulin Resistance and Chronic Diseases

Obesity (i.e., excess visceral fat) seems to promote insulin resistance via hormones and pro-inflammatory adipokines that compel cells to ignore insulin. Insulin levels build up, as do glucose levels, and the body's normal metabolism of molecular fats breaks down. Indirectly then, whatever causes obesity, which I believe to largely be the eating of easily digested carbohydrates, leads to insulin resistance. And as I wrote in the metabolic syndrome section, insulin resistance increases the risk of developing both heart disease and diabetes.

The old way of thinking rightly associated type 2 diabetes and obesity, but it wasn't until more research on insulin resistance was done that the central role insulin resistance (i.e., a poorly functioning glucose/insulin feedback system) plays in the development of diabetes became clear. The old way of thinking also blamed coronary heart disease squarely on fats, but that was rather incorrect. A concerted campaign based on misguided science compelled more Americans to eat more carbs, especially bad ones. But the obesity trend, along with diabetes and heart disease rates, got worse, not better. And as newer studies show, the science isn't clear on whether saturated fats increase people's risk of coronary heart disease.[48]

Insulin resistance better explains the development of coronary heart disease. Insulin resistance, encouraged by both obesity and eating easy-to-digest carbohydrates, makes the body metabolize fats in abnormal ways. In this environment, excess visceral fat will both make more triglycerides and release more free fatty acids (to be used for energy by other parts of the body). The liver turns these molecular fats into triglycerides, which it then releases into the blood. High triglycerides are strongly associated with increased risk of coronary disease and heart attacks.[49] Furthermore, a high-carbohydrate/low-fat diet seems to decrease HDL-cholesterol levels (which is bad), while a high-fat/low-carbohydrates diet seems to increase HDL-C (which is good) and lower triglyceride levels (also good).[50]

INCREASING AWARENESS

The paradigm shift to seeing chronic disease as being connected to insulin resistance (as being connected to easily digested carbs) is already happening in the public sphere. The L.A. Times in December 2010 quoted Dr. Willett, the chairman of Harvard's nutrition department, as saying, "[Dietary f]at is not the problem. If Americans could eliminate sugary beverages, potatoes, white bread, pasta, white rice and sugary snacks, we would wipe out almost all the problems we have with weight and diabetes and other metabolic diseases."[51] This wasn't a new insight for Dr. Willett. He wrote in his book published in 2001 that the best way to keep weight off is by eliminating simpler carbs, especially refined grains.[52] More evidence is being uncovered to support the hypothesis that refined carbohydrates lead to chronically elevated insulin (i.e., insulin resistance), which then leads to the buildup of excess visceral body fat.

That same L.A. Times article detailed a 2009 study showing that a diet high in saturated fats and low in carbohydrates had greater weight loss and better improvement in blood glucose, insulin, triglycerides, and cholesterol levels in a certain group.[53] Forty overweight or obese people with metabolic syndrome were put on one of two 1,500-calorie diets for 12 weeks. One diet was low-fat/high-carbohydrate, while the other was high-fat/low-carbohydrates. Notably, the saturated fats in the high-fat diet were three times the other diet, or in other words, 36 grams of saturated fats compared with 12 grams. Astonishingly, triglyceride levels fell by 50% and HDL-cholesterol levels went up by

47

15% in people on the high-fat diet.

How could this be? After all, the dogma on this issue is that a high-fat diet worsens people's cholesterol and fat levels. The study's authors theorized that when insulin is not high (i.e., when there is no insulin resistance) because there isn't much of a glucose load in a low-carb diet, molecular fats are not stored but rather burned (or oxidized) for energy by other cells. Thus, fat levels in the blood become lower.

A high-carb diet would, on the other hand, keep insulin levels high (i.e., maintain the insulin resistance), which would tell fat cells to store more fat (i.e., triglycerides), using raw material from what was eaten, mostly glucose, and to release free fatty acids into the blood, some of which the liver would make into triglycerides for the blood. This increase in the manufacture of bodily fat (as visceral fat grows bigger) and molecular fat (as fatty acids, cholesterols, and triglycerides) in the blood are all bad in terms of heart health. The role that certain diets play in relation to insulin has certainly become part of the new paradigm.

BASIC FOOD SCIENCE

Nothing would be more tiresome than eating and drinking if God had not made them a pleasure as well as a necessity.

– Voltaire

All food is made of molecules. We will concern ourselves with three kinds that are digested into our blood after they are broken down: fats, carbohydrates, and proteins. There are molecules our bodies can't digest, such as fiber. And yet there are other molecules that are digested and not a fat, carbohydrate, protein, or fiber: these include vitamins, minerals, and other phytonutrients that benefit our bodies.

DIETARY FATS

Fats come in all shapes and sizes and are made of carbon and hydrogen. The carbon backbones of some fats are long, while others are short. Some fats are saturated, meaning they have the maximum possible number of hydrogen atoms bound to their backbone, while other fats are unsaturated. These two properties define what a particular fat (such as lauric acid, a saturated fat, or omega-3 fatty acid, which is unsaturated) does in our bodies.

Trans Fats

Trans fats occur very rarely in nature. The vast majority of the trans fats a person will eat come from foods made using processed oils. These oils will have the words "hydrogenated" or "partially hydrogenated" on their labels. Food companies use oils containing trans fats to manufacture food products like cookies and frozen meals,

49

and restaurants use them to prepare dishes.

Because trans fats have not ever been a natural part of human diets, our bodies can't properly digest and metabolize them. Thus, it is better to avoid them. The mechanism is unclear, but there is no question that trans fats are more strongly associated with coronary heart disease than other fats (including saturated fats).[54]

Saturated Fats

Saturated fats are not all the same. Some are long-chain fats, and these are not quickly metabolized for energy. Thus, fat cells tend to collect them to make triglycerides (the stored form of fat). Medium and short-chain saturated fats, on the other hand, are burned for energy relatively quickly and thus don't promote the growth of body fat.

Lauric acid, found in coconut oil, is an example of such a medium-chain saturated fat. Short-chain saturated fats tend to be in fermented dairy products like *dahi* (yogurt) and pickles and made by anaerobic bacteria in the colon. As a whole, saturated fats are less harmful than trans fats. Some saturated fats aren't harmful at all. This causes results from various studies on saturated fats to go against the dogma that saturated fats are bad for the heart.

Consider a meta-analysis involving almost 350,000 people. Some reviewed studies revealed a correlation between high-saturated fats and more coronary heart disease was found, but just as many did not. According to the authors, there was "no significant evidence for concluding that dietary saturated fat is associated with an increased risk of CHD or CVD [coronary heart disease or cardiovascular disease, which includes strokes]."[55] Note, this meta-analysis was funded in part by the National Dairy Council, a group interested in showing saturated fats in a good light.

Let's look at studies not funded by corporations making similar conclusions. A 1981 study on two Polynesian groups concluded that the group that ate more coconut oil (made almost entirely of saturated fats) experienced no more incidences of heart disease than the group that had little saturated fat in their diet.[56] A 2004 study of 235 postmenopausal women concluded that a diet with higher saturated fat content led to *less* coronary artery narrowing (based on what physicians saw during coronary angiography) compared with women on a higher carbohydrate diet with little saturated fats.[57]

A 1967 epidemiological study among Indian railway workers showed that those in north India had much less heart disease than those living in the south.[58] The authors hypothesized that there was something protective about the short-chain saturated fats prevalent in the northern diet (from the high consumption of milk and fermented dairies), or something harmful about the long-chain poly*un*saturated fats found in seed oils, which were heavily used in South India.

Finally, the strongest evidence comes from a 2009 meta-analysis of 146 prospective cohort studies and 43 randomized controlled trials (RCTs provide the strongest evidence in clinical research) from the 1950s to 2007. The researchers found that a diet high in *saturated* fats did *not* lead to more coronary heart disease.[59] Instead, what led to more coronary disease (and risk factors for coronary disease) were diets (1) high in trans fats and (2) high in foods with a high glycemic index such as sugar and refined grains

The 1967 epidemiological study done in India may hint that using seed oils for cooking may be harmful. Because saturated fats have the maximum number of hydrogen atoms possible, they are less likely to form free radicals (which are bad) when heated for cooking compared with *un*saturated fats that are prevalent in seed and other plant oils. Thus, saturated fat-dense foods like *ghee* (clarified butter) and coconut oil are better than olive oil (a mostly *un*saturated fat made popular because of the Mediterranean diet) for cooking.

So what is the bottom line with saturated fats? One, they are ideal for cooking purposes. Two, eating a moderate amount of saturated fats will not harm you. As Dr. Robert Eckel, former president of the AHA, said in response to the 2009 meta-analysis, said, "No one is saying that some saturated fat is going to harm you."[60]

Unsaturated Fats: Mono- and Polyunsaturated Fats

*Un*saturated fats are missing hydrogen atoms on their carbon backbones. Vegetable oils like corn, safflower, olive, and canola oils are rich in unsaturated fats (though they are mostly *poly*unsaturated in corn and safflower oils and more *mono*unsaturated in olive and canola oils). Unsaturated fats are also abundant in nuts, seeds, and avocados.

The Harvard School of Public Health states that *un*saturated fats "improve blood cholesterol levels, ease inflammation, stabilize heart rhythms," citing two trials that compared consumption of unsaturated fats with consumption of carbohydrates (which had adverse effects).[61] Seemingly, these benefits seem most associated with omega-3 fatty acids, a kind of polyunsaturated fat, and olive oil, rich in a monounsaturated fat named oleic acid (and phenols).

Like any fat, unsaturated fats are good in moderate amounts. Your body's cells need a broad variety of molecular fats to function, but apply caution when using oils containing mostly *un*saturated fats for cooking. Because of their chemistry, unsaturated fats are less cohesive than saturated fats.

Take note that foods dense in saturated fats like butter, *ghee*, and coconut oil are solid at room temperature, while olive, canola, and corn oils, among other plant and seed oils dense in *un*saturated fats, are liquid. Because they are less cohesive, *un*saturated fats tend to be more unstable when heated for cooking. *Un*saturated fats are thus more likely to become oxidized under that heat and produce free radicals, which are then transferred into your food and body.

Omega-3 and 6 Fatty Acids

Omega-3 fatty acid is the most popular fat today. It's a long-chain *poly*unsaturated fat that helps by reducing the general level of inflammation. Like fats in general, it integrates into cellular membranes. Omega-3 fat is also essential for the normal development of a child's brain and other tissues. Studies show that it likely helps keep adult brains and hearts healthy, which is why health experts tell people to eat fatty fish (e.g., salmon), chia (or Salvia), grounded flaxseed, or walnuts.[62] Evidence suggests that replacing saturated fats with polyunsaturated fats like omega-3 and -6 fatty acids can lower your risk of coronary heart disease.[63]

Omega-6 fatty acid is a related long-chain *poly*unsaturated fat common in corn and other vegetable oils. It is also essential for proper development. But in adults, omega-6 fats tend to become eicosanoids (e.g., thromboxanes, prostacyclins, and leukotrienes), which trigger inflammation.[64] (Omega-3 fatty acids also become eicosanoids, but more slowly.) Some experts believe that when the body unnecessarily produces eicosanoids, it gives rise to inflammatory diseases like asthma and lupus. A higher than normal level of inflammation also encourages the development of chronic diseases.

Why Some Oils are Bad for Cooking

Free radicals are molecules produced from oxidation that will themselves oxidize other molecules. They are believed to cause, or at least promote, chronic diseases. Oxidation doesn't happen just in the heating process. When oil is squeezed from seeds or plants, the elements of heat, light, and oxygen begin to oxidize the oil. The more processing oil goes through before making it into a bottle, the more of it will be oxidized. This is why health buffs demand cold-pressed oils in dark glass bottles without added preservatives.

Generally, oils with lots of mono*un*saturated fats (e.g., olive and canola oils) tend not to become free radicals while oils with lots of poly*un*saturated fats (e.g., safflower and sunflower oils) do become free radicals thanks to their chemical properties.[65] Note, however, that cold-pressed (i.e., unrefined) oils, including extra-virgin olive oil, have lower smoke points. This makes them less ideal for cooking, as they break down at high temperatures. This is why health experts tell people not to use extra-virgin olive oil for cooking. Canola oil is better because it has a smoking-point temperature of 400°F and is thus less likely to break down during high-temperature cooking.

Saturated fat-dense foods like butter, *ghee*, and coconut oil are also good for cooking, but in medium-heat cooking. This is in comparison to canola oil, which is ideal for high-heat cooking, and corn oil, which is ideal for deep-frying, as it has a smoking point temperature of 450°F. Those oils are ideal in those settings because they won't break down at those temperatures. Because of the nature of their chemical bonds, saturated fats tend to not become free radicals like many plant oils do from the basic elements of nature.[66]

Cholesterol

Half a century ago, scientists discovered that blood cholesterol was linked to heart disease. You probably know from a few visits to the doctor that high total cholesterol is bad – as is high LDL-C – but that high HDL-C is good. This is why you have been told to avoid cholesterol in your diet. But for most people, *dietary* cholesterol doesn't affect the level of *blood* cholesterol very much.

First, cholesterol is not a fat molecule but a fatty steroid needed for cell membranes. Your body makes 80% of the cholesterol needed by your cells; meaning 20% comes from what you eat. If you happen to eat a lot of cholesterol one day (e.g., you eat 4 egg yolks), your body will simply make less cholesterol to keep the total cholesterol for the day balanced.

According to the Harvard School of Public Health, *blood* cholesterol for some people is influenced much more than expected by how much cholesterol that person eats. Their website says, "For these 'responders,' avoiding cholesterol-rich foods can have a substantial effect on blood cholesterol levels. Unfortunately, at this point there is no way other than by trial and error to identify responders from non-responders to dietary cholesterol."[67] But for most people, the amount of cholesterol they eat doesn't change the level of cholesterol in their blood very much.

CARBOHYDRATES

Carbohydrates are made of carbon, hydrogen, and oxygen atoms and commonly categorized as simple and complex. Mono- and disaccharides are simple carbohydrates and include sugars. Oligo- and polysaccharides are complex carbohydrates. Nutritionists long considered complex carbohydrates good for you because they were digested slowly, but this isn't true. Starches, such as what is found in potatoes and the endosperm of all grains are oligosaccharides and quickly digested. Cellulose is a polysaccharide, which isn't digestible; polysaccharides tend to be fiber.

Sugars

Sugars are mono- and disaccharides and thus considered simple carbohydrates. Table sugar (i.e., sucrose) is made of two monosaccharides, glucose and fructose. High Fructose Corn Syrup (HFCS) is similar, but some glucose is artificially made into fructose. Table sugar and HFCS are quickly and easily digested by your body. Some experts believe the heavy use by food companies of HFCS, as opposed to table sugar, is the biggest culprit behind the obesity epidemic.

Glucose, a monosaccharide component of table sugar and HFCS, is by nature the most readily available and usable form of energy. It is the only carbohydrate the pancreas senses before releasing insulin into the blood. Fructose, in contrast, does not cause a rise in insulin. Also, unlike glucose, which is used by the vast majority of cells, only liver cells use fructose. When liver cells become saturated with carbohydrates, which happens from a high-carb diet or by insulin resistance or diabetes, they make triglycerides from fructose and send them to fat cells for storage.[68]

Glucose is also made into triglycerides, especially when insulin levels are high (i.e., due to a high-carbohydrate diet, insulin resistance, or diabetes). High blood glucose levels cause high insulin levels. This tells visceral fat cells to take glucose, use some for energy, and convert some to glycerol, the backbone of triglycerides. Some glucose becomes free fatty acids in other cells, which are combined with glycerol to make triglyceride molecules.) The more insulin spikes there are, the more fat molecules are accumulated into visceral fat, causing the tissues to grow.

This is how simple carbs like table sugar and HFCS are linked to body fat and insulin resistance. A 2010 meta-analysis showed that these carbohydrates, not fats, are linked to an increased risk of heart disease. The authors thus urged people to eat less sugars, starches, and refined grains, which are foods with the highest Glycemic Index numbers.[69]

Glycemic Index and Glycemic Load

Instead of looking at carbohydrates as simple or complex, it is more useful to think of them as high or low Glycemic Load carbohydrates. First, let me explain the Glycemic Index (GI). The GI concept was developed by a University of Sydney group and assigns a number to a particular food to describe how *quickly* the carbohydrates in that food become blood glucose. The lower a food's GI is, the less quickly one's blood glucose will rise. Connecting the dots, the lower a food's GI, the less insulin will be required from the pancreas. Therefore, the GI describes the quality of carbohydrates in a useful way. In general, it is easier for you to control your blood glucose and insulin levels when you eat mostly foods with low GI. This is true also for people with diabetes.

Vegetables and fruit are carbohydrate-dense, but because they are mostly water and contain fiber, which slows the digestion of carbohydrates, they tend have low GIs. In other words, eating a vegetable or most (but not all) fruits does not increase blood glucose or insulin levels quickly. For comparison, refined grains – which are the starchy endosperm without the fiber found in natural whole grains – have high GIs. Refined grains thus tend to elevate blood glucose and insulin quickly. The bottom line on GI is that lower GI foods are better for the body, especially the glucose/insulin feedback system.

Harvard researchers developed an advanced version of the GI concept called the Glycemic Load (GL). The GL is more realistic in describing how a food will affect your blood glucose and insulin levels. Whereas a food's GI tells us how quickly blood glucose rises, a food's GL better tells both how quickly and by how much our blood glucose rise, and it is based on the amount of carbohydrates found in that food's typical serving size. Still, the same principle applies to GL: the lower it is, the better it is for the body. And accordingly, vegetables and most fruits as well as fiber-rich grain cereals have low GLs, while sugars and refined grains have high GLs.

The table below lists GLs (Glycemic Loads) for common Indian foods.[70] These GLs came from people with mild insulin resistance (i.e., mild impaired glucose tolerance), and I used it because the list was far more extensive than that from healthy people. The main purpose of this table is to give you a general idea of a food's GL relative to other foods.

Food or Dish	Glycemic Index	Serving Size	Glycemic Load
Appam (thin pancake made from fermented rice flour batter with tender coconut) eaten with Bengal gram curry†	90	250 g	58
Bajra (*Penniseteum typhoideum*), eaten as roasted bread made from bajra flour	55	75 g (dry)	28
Chapatti, wheat flour, thin, with green gram (*Phaseolus aureus*) dhal	81	200 g	41
Dhokla, leavened, fermented, steamed cake; dehusked chickpea and wheat semolina	31	150 g	9
Dosai (parboiled and raw rice, soaked, ground, fermented and fried) with chutney	77	150 g	30
Idli (parboiled and raw rice + black dhal, soaked, ground, fermented, steamed) with chutney	77	250 g	40
Jowar, roasted bread made from Jowar flour (*Sorghum vulgare*)	77	70 g (dry)	39
Millet/Ragi (*Eleucine coracana*) flour eaten as roasted bread	104	70 g (dry)	52
Pongal (rice and roasted green gram dhal, pressure cooked)	90	250 g	47
Poori (deep-fried wheat flour dough) with potato palya (mashed potato)	82	150 g	34
Puttu (rice flour, steamed with tender coconut) eaten with	79	250 g	58

Food or Dish	Glycemic Index	Serving Size	Glycemic Load
Bengal gram curry			
Semolina (*Triticum aestivum*) with fermented black gram dhal (*Phaseolus mungo*)	46	71 g (dry)	23
Upittu (roasted semolina and onions, cooked in water)	67	150 g	28
Uppuma kedgeree (millet, legumes, fenugreek seeds; roasted and cooked in water)	19	150 g	6

The table below contains GLs for other common foods eaten in the U.S. and other developed parts of the world.

Food or Dish	Glycemic Index	Serving Size	Glycemic Load
Brown (Oryza Sativa), boiled (South India)	50	150 g	17
Milled (white), high amylose (IR42) rice, boiled 22 min (Philippines)	59	150 g	25
Ice cream, NS (USA)	62	50 g	7
White bread with butter (Canada)	84	100 g	28
Chickpeas, curry, canned (Canasia Foods Ltd., Scarborough, Canada)	41	150 g	7
Lentils, type NS (USA)	28	150 g	5
Kidney beans (Canada)	46	150 g	11
Peas, dried, boiled (Australia)	22	150 g	2
Apple, NS (USA)	40	120 g	6
Banana, ripe (all yellow) (USA)	51	120 g	13
Mango, ripe (*Mangifera indica*) (India)	60	120 g	9
Oranges (Sunkist, Van Nuys, CA, USA)	48	120 g	5
Orange juice, reconstituted from frozen concentrate (USA)	57	250 ml	15
Taco shells, cornmeal-based, baked (Old El Paso Foods Co., Toronto, Canada)	68	20 g	8
Pizza, cheese (Pillsbury Canada Ltd., Toronto, Canada)	60	100 g	16

Food or Dish	Glycemic Index	Serving Size	Glycemic Load
Peanuts (Canada)	13	50 g	1
Spaghetti, homemade, durum wheat, no monoglyceride, boiled 6 min (Denmark)	59	180 g	28
Corn chips, Nachips™ (Old El Paso Foods Co., Canada)	74	50 g	21
Clif bar, Cookies & Cream flavor (Clif Bar Inc, Berkeley, CA, USA)	101	65 g	49
Black Bean soup (Wil-Pack Foods, San Pedro, CA, USA)	64	250 g	17
Carrots, NS (Canada)	92	80 g	6
Russet, baked without fat (USA)	94	150 g	28
Sweet potato, NS (Canada)	48	150 g	16

Some experts say a rule of thumb is that foods with a GL of 10 or less are good because they don't affect your glucose or insulin very much. Foods with GL of 20 or greater are bad in terms of how they affect your glucose and insulin levels.

In general, to keep your blood glucose/insulin feedback system in good working order, eat more foods that are low to medium (10 to 20) on the GL scale (e.g., vegetables, fruits, legumes, and whole grains), and fewer of the high GL foods (e.g., refined grains, junk food, and sugars). Note, low to medium GL foods are beneficial beyond just having a minimal impact on blood glucose and insulin levels: they tend to be full of vitamins, minerals, phytonutrients, and fiber.

Fiber

Fibers are carbohydrates in food that can't be digested. Stomach acid, bile, and enzymes can't break down fiber the way they break down most carbs, fats, and proteins (into monosaccharides, fatty acids, and amino acids, respectively). Nutritionists classify fiber, found in plants and not in meat, as soluble or insoluble.

Plants contain both kinds of fiber to varying degrees. An apple has soluble fiber in its flesh, but *in*soluble fiber in its skin. That said, plants tend to be denser in one kind of fiber. Whole grains have more *in*soluble fiber, while fibers in legumes are mostly soluble. The distinction is important because they do different things in the body.

Soluble fiber

Fibers in the following foods are mostly soluble: legumes (*dals* and beans); oats and barley; fruits like plums, berries, bananas, and apples; vegetables like broccoli and carrots; root vegetables like sweet potatoes and onions; and psyllium seed husk, a common laxative. Soluble fiber becomes a sticky gelatinous substance in the intestines. This sticky stuff holds on to easily digested carbohydrates, making them slower to absorb into the body.[vii]

Soluble fiber then reduces the speed with which carbohydrates, even the amounts of carbohydrates, get digested. This reduces the level of the insulin spikes from the pancreas in response to what carbohydrates make it into the blood. This is probably why a regular diet high in soluble fiber is associated with a lower risk of developing diabetes.[71]

A regular diet high in soluble fiber also helps people with diabetes, improving their control of blood glucose levels.[72] Additionally, soluble fiber keeps cholesterol levels lower by the same principle, grabbing cholesterol-rich bile acids and holding them until they pass out of the intestines.

While your body cannot digest soluble fiber, anaerobic gut bacteria can. They turn much of the soluble fiber into short-chain fatty acids, which evidence shows benefit the colon by providing cells with energy, and they may help lower free fatty acids floating in the blood.[73] This is likely why legumes like *dal* have been considered good for the digestive tract since antiquity, being held in high-esteem by the Ayurvedic practitioners of ancient India.

Insoluble fiber

Fibers in the following foods are mostly *in*soluble: whole grains and pure bran; nuts and seeds like flaxseed; vegetables like green beans,

---

[vii] The presence of soluble fiber is why most fruits have low GIs and GLs despite having lots of glucose.

cauliflower, zucchini, and celery; and the skin of many fruits including plums and tomatoes. Unlike soluble fiber, which dissolves and becomes a sticky substance, *in*soluble fiber does not dissolve in water and thus makes stool bulkier and softer, thus easing its transit from the digestive tract.

Insoluble fiber is also good for heart health. A study of almost 44,000 U.S. men over 6 years found that men who ate 10 grams or more fiber daily from breakfast cereal (where the fiber is mostly *in*soluble) had a 19% lower risk of suffering a heart attack compared with men who did not.[74]

Lower risks of heart attack were also seen among men who ate 10 grams more fiber per day where the fiber came from fruits or vegetables, but the reduction in risk was greater when the fiber came from grain cereal, which is mostly *in*soluble. There is also evidence that *in*soluble fiber, like soluble fiber, reduces the risk of developing diabetes, particularly *in*soluble fiber from whole grain cereal.[75] This is why experts tell people to eat more whole grains.

PROTEINS

Admittedly, I give proteins short shrift in this section. This is because they are the least controversial component of food from the perspective of human health. Proteins provide amino acids, the basic building blocks of all cells.

Eight amino acids are considered essential because they aren't produced by the body but are necessary for proper growth, development, and maintenance of life. The remaining amino acids, the *un*essential amino acids, are also necessary for life but can be made by your body.

In general, eggs and meat (technically, muscle meat) contain all 8 essential amino acids that your body cannot make.[76] This is why they are called sources of high-quality protein. In contrast, an individual plant food will not have all of these amino acids. But combining legumes (which are low in an amino acid called methionine) and grains (low in lysine) in a single meal, like a typical Indian meal made of *channa* (chickpeas) and *parathas* (leavened whole wheat), will provide you with all 8 essential amino acids.[77]

Allow me to quickly illustrate how some sources of protein may be good while others are bad. A 2007 survey from a National Cancer Institute cohort of about 500,000 older Americans found "strong evidence that people who eat a lot of red [in this study, beef, pork, and lamb] and processed meats [e.g., bacon, ham, and sausages] have greater risk of developing colorectal and lung cancer than do people who eat small quantities."[78] Red and processed meats have also been implicated, though with weaker evidence, in the development of coronary heart disease. What is certain is that protein-dense plant foods like legumes (like *dal*) and tree nuts have, on the other hand, not been associated with cancer or other chronic diseases.

PHYTONUTRIENTS

Phytonutrients are not one of the three components of food, but rather they are naturally occurring compounds found only in plants that interact with cells in your body. There are hundreds to thousands of phytonutrients in the plants we eat, but modern science has illuminated the roles of only a few. Phytonutrients are widely believed to be beneficial for your health.

The first phytonutrients isolated in labs and studied were what we today call vitamins. Their role in human health is clear. Vitamin deficiency leads to debilitating disease like rickets, a bone disorder caused by vitamin D deficiency, and beriberi, a vitamin B1-deficiency disease studied by Dr. McCarrison in colonial India. Beta-carotene, found in orange-colored plants like mangoes, papayas, and carrots, as well as leafy greens like spinach and kale, is a precursor for vitamin A, the deficiency of which causes night blindness.

Another set of phytonutrients are antioxidants, some of which are vitamins that capture and neutralize free radicals and thus prevent other molecules in the body from being oxidized. Antioxidants don't seem to work in isolation (e.g., taking only vitamin E), but do seem to work when eaten in their natural forms (e.g., in fruits and vegetables that contain vitamin E) to prevent numerous diseases including heart disease and cancers.[79]

Recently described phytonutrients show they may reduce the risk of some chronic diseases. Lycopenes in tomatoes appear to reduce the risk of developing prostate cancer.[80] Edible plants are full of minerals like potassium and magnesium, which have been shown to control blood pressure and heart rhythms. People for years believed eating lots of fiber would lower their risk of developing colon cancer, but recent better-designed studies with more subjects have shown this isn't so.[81]

High daily amounts of fibers alone didn't reduce the risk of colon cancer, but regular consumption of foods where fiber is plentiful, namely a diet with lots of vegetables and fruits, is linked to lower incidences of cancers and other chronic diseases (as I described above). Some researchers believe this effect is likely due to phytonutrients in these foods. A healthy Indian diet, being based on plants and having plenty of phytonutrients, probably offers similar benefits.

PART II

THE HEALTHY

INDIAN DIET

WHAT ARE DIETS

Our bodies are our gardens, to which our wills are gardeners.

– William Shakespeare

PEOPLE'S DIETS ARE FUNDAMENTALLY PATTERNS OF FOODS

In the following pages, I will describe a pattern of foods constituting a regular diet that is both Indian in nature and also healthy. To get the most out of reading this book, *you* must ultimately select foods that you like and fit the profile of the healthy Indian diet. I keep the definition of the healthy Indian diet fairly general. You will not catch me saying, "Eat more red *dal*," but you will catch me describing why *dals* and other legumes are good for you. Ultimately, I want you to pick and choose what legumes and other foods are to your liking. The only way you will adopt healthy Indian meals over the long term is if you find these meals tasty.

I keep the advice general for another reason. I don't believe any diet completely prevents disease. No specific set of foods eaten every day is a magic bullet. After all, we haven't ever been able to fully control our food supply, environment, or the genes we are born with. Our diets, no matter how healthy, can't make up for all the potential problems, big and small, in our environments and genes. Yet, all things considered, our diets can influence our general state of health and improve our chances, sometimes dramatically, of having a better quality of life well into old age.

The third reason I keep the advice general is to convey the idea that the sum of the parts is better than all the parts in isolation. There are all kinds of synergies in nature, and thus in traditional diets, that science doesn't fully understand. This synergy is best demonstrated by pondering these two observations:

(1) A daily multivitamin does not reduce the risk of chronic diseases, and

(2) Plant-based diets, which contain the same vitamins but usually in smaller amounts as well as other phytonutrients, are associated with lower risks of heart disease, diabetes, and some cancers.[82,83]

Some diets have a magic-like effect on the body. The modified Atkins diet, which is a low-carbohydrate, high-fat diet, can help many people lose an incredible amount of weight quickly. The high-natural carbohydrate Ornish diet, when coupled with intense lifestyle changes, can reverse atherosclerosis. My desire is to describe a healthy diet that is different in philosophy to the Atkins and Ornish diets in that the healthy Indian diet can be followed every day, where your body gets all the nutrients it needs, and offers health benefits without making any dramatic changes to your lifestyle (though I do encourage exercise, yoga, meditation, and socializing).

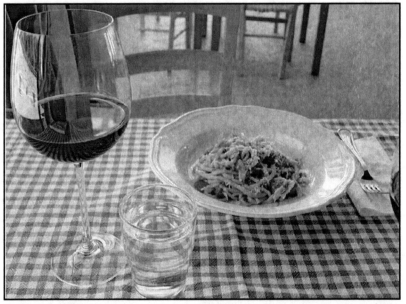

Figure 7: Whole grain pasta, vegetables and wine are parts of the traditional Mediterranean Diet. (Photo used under Creative Commons from roblisameehan.)

MEDITERRANEAN DIET

The Mediterranean diet is the best comparison to the diet I describe in this book. Like the healthy Indian diet, the Mediterranean diet is based on traditional combinations of foods, mostly plant foods, and tastes good. And it is a healthy diet. You have probably heard that eating dishes from the Mediterranean diet will help your heart stay healthy. Lots of scientific research supports the healthiness of the diet, even in patients who have suffered a heart attack or have Alzheimer's dementia.[84,85]

And like the healthy Indian diet, there was no such thing as the Mediterranean diet in the real world until very recently. The diet is basically a pattern of foods based on what people in the cities, islands, and countries surrounding the Mediterranean Sea have been eating traditionally for millennia. In other words, the Mediterranean diet is a modern construct that conveys a health pattern of eating. Below are guidelines for what makes the Mediterranean diet according to the AHA.[86]

- High consumption of fruits, vegetables, bread and other cereals, potatoes, beans, nuts and seeds
- Olive oil is an important monounsaturated fat source
- Dairy products, fish and poultry are consumed in low to moderate amounts, and little red meat is eaten
- Eggs are consumed zero to four times a week
- Wine is consumed in low to moderate amounts

Although people in the Mediterranean don't eat a Mediterranean diet per se, Italians having a traditional (not modern) diet will eat the same kinds of foods that people in Morocco eat, although the preparation will differ. A main part of the diet, olive oil, is used by people in Italy, Morocco, Spain, Egypt, Greece, Israel, Lebanon, and Turkey. So though people in different parts of Italy (or any Mediterranean country) eat different dishes, the foundational foods in those dishes are the same: olive oil, fish, fresh vegetables, wine, and so on. Notably, the Mediterranean diet makes little to no use of red meat or refined grains.

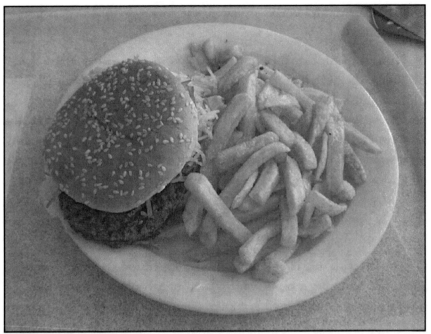

Figure 8: White bread, red meat, and fried potatoes are part of the typical Modern Diet. (Photo used under Creative Commons from Like the Grand Canyon.)

WESTERN OR MODERN DIET

The diet that was once called "Western" and blamed for the epidemics of chronic disease is now often called the "Modern" diet. The Modern diet is commonly eaten in big cities around the world, from Rio de Janeiro to Moscow, from Beijing to Mumbai, not just in the U.S. and Europe thanks to two trends. First, globalization has made more people in underdeveloped parts of the world richer, and they are demanding more foods like meat. This has also made it easier for companies needing new markets to sell their products in emerging economies. Second, industrialization has encouraged food companies to make food that is cheaper and lasts longer, which means natural foods go through more processing and more chemicals are added to them in order to sell as much as possible. These trends are not new, as observations of Pima Indians in the American Southwest around the 1850s and "Bengali gentlemen" under the British Raj in the early

69

1900s illustrate. McDonald's may be the most obvious beneficiary of these modern trends.

However, McDonald's and other companies that have taken advantage of these trends, to the detriment of people's health I must add, are not solely to blame. After all, just like Americans during the post-war period, people in emerging nations want to adopt the Western diet because it may taste better and because it conveys status. Meanwhile, Indians and other immigrants who came to the U.S. and other developed countries, just like Americans and other Westerners, had little choice but to adopt what foods were available locally. Consider also that people in the West didn't know until recently just how harmful Modern diets were.

The Modern diet is based on three kinds of foods. First are refined grains like hamburger buns, white rice, flour, cookies, chips, which are rich in simple (sugars) and complex (starches) carbohydrates that are easy to digest. I made the case earlier how these kinds of carbohydrates are linked to insulin resistance as well diabetes and heart disease.

Second are foods containing trans fats, namely margarine and partially hydrogenated vegetable oils. People don't use these at home, but many restaurants still do. And no fat has been so strongly linked to coronary disease and heart attacks like trans fats. Third are red meat and processed meat. It is not entirely clear whether the meat itself, the processing, or the cooking is to blame, but both have been linked to increasing risks of cancers. Let me summarize the foundations of the Modern diet.

- Refined carbohydrates
- Foods containing trans fats
- Red and processed meat
- Low consumption of plant foods

The Modern diet has harmful foods and not enough plant foods, where much of the vitamins, minerals, fiber, and other phytonutrients that our bodies need can be found.

HEALTHY INDIAN DIET

Historically speaking, nutrition researchers and physicians who had the right resources did not study Indian diets in the same way they studied American and European diets since the 1950s. This situation has improved recently, and discoveries about elements of different Indian diets are coming to light.

The healthy Indian diet I describe is based on traditional cuisines and is reversed-engineered from what we know thanks to modern science (e.g., eating brown rice regularly helps to reduce the risk of developing diabetes, while eating white rice raises it). Many times, tradition and what experts advise based on science overlap. For example, people in India traditionally ate brown and wild rice; white rice, as doctors in colonial Indian pointed out, was an adoption of Modern diets.

In crafting a healthy Indian diet, I considered what foods, traditionally speaking, are common in all parts of the Indian subcontinent. The most obvious element is spices. Since ancient times, India has been known for spices. Ayurvedic practitioners prescribed combinations of spices to help people get better, and this way of thinking made it into daily cooking. Spices are a unique cultural heritage for all Indian people, and although the spice mix used differs between Gujarat and Andhra Pradesh, or Bengal and Himachal Pradesh, they are made of the same spices: asafetida, cumin, black peppercorn, red chili pepper, cinnamon, cloves, turmeric, and so on.

One foundation of all Indian diets is the emphasis on plant foods, another is that everyone eats *dals* and other legumes, and to varying extents fermented dairy products like *dahi* and pickles. These basic similarities constitute the healthy Indian diet. Here are the foundations of the healthy Indian diet.

- High consumption of vegetables and some fruits
- Spices are used in all dishes
- Legumes are consumed regularly with whole grains for complete proteins

- Fermented dairy products and pickles are eaten often
- Meats are consumed in low quantities
- Very low consumption of refined grains and sugars

There you have it! These are the only guidelines you will ever need to craft your own healthy Indian diet, or simply healthy Indian dishes.

I will explain in the rest of this book why these foundational foods make the Indian diet healthy. Importantly, I will explain for those of you who eat Indian food regularly what can be added to the typical Indian diet to make it better for you, and what should be reduced or dropped altogether.

USEFUL PHILOSOPHIES FOR THE HEALTHY INDIAN DIET

Perfection is the Enemy of the Good

The philosopher Voltaire wrote this line in a poem, *"le mieux est l'ennemi du bien."* This has come to mean that perfection is the enemy of the good, which is commonly interpreted as meaning "don't try to be perfect when you start something new." Trying to be perfect may get in the way of becoming good or competent. Discipline is definitely necessary to make positive changes, but focus your discipline on action and not results. Be aware that when trying to do something, like adopting a healthier diet, you will fail in some ways. No transformation is smooth, so cut yourself some slack.

When adopting elements of the healthy Indian diet, give yourself some leeway to cheat on some days. If you crave something you decided to stop eating, go and have it – but only on occasion. I for one, even years after changing to brown rice, eat white rice occasionally. But as long as you try honestly to eat well most of the time, and actually do so for most meals during the week, be satisfied with that.

Moderation in All Things

After experiencing *nirvana*, the Buddha began preaching a philosophy called *madhyama-pratipad* or "the Middle Way." This approach advocates moderation in all things. Although the Buddha preached his philosophy as a way of life, speaking on the balance between earthly, sensual pleasures and self-suffering in the search of truth, I believe it can also be applied to your way of eating.

You should not feel like you must completely restrict a certain food, unless you wish to of course. The main point is that too much of something is often bad. Clearly, eating too much of a savory snack like potato chips is bad, but eating too much leafy greens at the exclusion of other foods like fruits or *dals* can also be bad. Eating all foods in moderation provides your body with the broad nutrition it needs for an optimal state of well-being.

A theory called "hormesis" describes the phenomenon where too much of a particular thing is toxic, but a little bit does some good. Alcohol, for example, shows an increased life expectancy in people who drink two to three such beverages daily. More than that amount has been shown to lower life expectancy, but drinking no alcohol at all, interestingly, also lowers life expectancy.

The hormesis effect has been demonstrated with low-level radiation too and may be applicable to food, although nobody knows. Perhaps a couple of scoops of ice cream every couple of nights may provide an immeasurable benefit, whereas too much may do some harm. Anyway, hormesis does illuminate the benefit of things in moderation, including what you eat.

Focus on Changing your Environment, not your Behavior

Changing your environment is easier than changing your behavior. This may explain why most people can't stick to a new fad diet for long, whether or not they see the results. It simply takes too much willpower to sustain such changes to what are ingrained, automatic habits. Also, some foods, especially sugars, are addictive and give the same dopamine rush as other addictions. Thus, focusing on changing what you *do* "cold turkey" is noble but often misguided.

You will have greater success by changing your environment and then trying to change your behavior in the new context. For example,

73

move whatever you want to stop eating from the kitchen countertop, where it is in full view, to the pantry and away from plain sight. Likewise, put something you want to eat more of on the countertop. This will help you change your diet because it makes it easier on your willpower to avoid what you know you shouldn't eat and makes it easier to eat or cook more of what you consciously want to.

Basic Principles of the Healthy Indian Diet

1. Base your diet on plant foods like leafy greens and fruits. They are rich in vitamins, minerals, fiber, antioxidants, and anti-inflammatory phytonutrients that help the body keep inflammation and insulin levels normal.

2. Cut out trans fats such as those found in partially or fully hydrogenated oils.

3. Cook using moderate amounts of foods rich in saturated fats like *ghee* and coconut oil.

4. Have legumes like *dal* and protein-dense tree nuts regularly. Combine them with whole grains to get complete proteins.

5. Fill your dishes with spices, especially turmeric, ginger, garlic, and peppers.

6. Remove refined grains like white rice and bread, finely ground flour, and table sugar. They offer the body easily digestible carbohydrates and nearly zero nutrition. This also means do not eat too many starchy foods like white potatoes.

7. Have whole grains like brown rice and coarsely ground grains like millet and sorghum. They offer the body abundant nutrition and fiber.

8. Include fermented foods like yogurts (*dahi* and *curds*) and pickles regularly.

9. Create a daily diet that is varied and, above all else, tasty.

Follow these basic principles, and you will have yourself a healthy Indian diet. You will provide your body with the proper nutrition it

75

needs, and thus you will improve your chances against becoming obese or developing heart disease, diabetes, and some cancers. You will also feel well, mentally sharper, and outwardly more beautiful, benefiting from whole foods found in nature and the wisdom found in traditional Indian cooking.

FOUNDATIONS OF THE HEALTHY INDIAN DIET

MOSTLY PLANTS

> *Eat food. Not too much. Mostly plants.*
>
> – Michael Pollan

That is the best advice I have read on how to eat healthily. By the word "food," journalist Michael Pollan means natural or whole foods, not processed or refined food products. By saying "not too much," he reinforces the wisdom that our portions need to be reasonable. His final sentence captures the point I will make here: that a healthy Indian diet is mostly plants.

Fortunately, not only are most Indian dishes made of plants, each with its own unique texture and flavor, these dishes are also spicy, peppery, savory, pungent, sour, sweet, and earthy. You can definitely taste the individual vegetables that go into *subzis*, from delectable asparagus (for the *subzi*, go to page 128) to hearty butternut squash (for a recipe of this with black chickpeas, go to page 130), but you will taste more of the spices they are cooked with. The taste of *palak paneer* (page 126) and other dishes are less influenced by spices on the other hand and more defined by the vegetable themselves, or in this case by rich cream. You will find other mostly plant dishes in Part III.

The Case for Mostly Plants

The typical Indian diet is mostly plants. Throughout history, Hindus in general have been vegetarian, as have Jains. The many Hindu cuisines influenced the typical Indian diet more than other ways of cooking. Despite waves of meat-eating peoples coming to the Subcontinent and settling there, plants remained the base of all Indian cuisines. Even in meat dishes had by Sikhs, Muslims, Christians, and some Hindus, there are plenty of vegetables and spices.

Therefore, I have no need to argue why the healthy Indian diet is plant-based, it has simply always been this way. Let me explain why a mostly plant diet is healthy. Dr. Willet of Harvard, a luminary in nutrition and health, made a compelling case for why plants are good. In his book "Eat, Drink, and Be Healthy," he admits that plants are *not* a cure-all and discusses conflicting reports on whether eating fresh fruits and vegetables help reduce the risk of cancers. Still, he is convinced that they do far more good for human health than any other food.

Based on a review of hundreds of studies by the International Association for Research on Cancer, Dr. Willet stated that eating a lot of fruits *probably* reduces the risk of the following cancers: lung, stomach, and esophageal cancers. Such a diet *may* also reduce the risk of colon, kidney, bladder, ovarian, mouth, and throat cancers. As for vegetables, eating a lot of them *probably* reduces the risk of colon and esophageal cancers and *may* reduce the risk of lung, kidney, ovarian, stomach, mouth, and throat cancers.

Other studies show a diet of mostly plants helps prevent other chronic diseases and ensures a longer, better quality of life. A study of 5,600 Italians at least 60 years old showed that the group eating an "Olive Oil & Vegetables" diet had the best health based on a number of parameters.[87] This group also had the lowest death rate.

A larger observational study of 12,700 middle-aged men in seven countries, including the United States, Greece, and Japan, demonstrated that vegetable-based diets were associated with a lower risk of coronary heart disease.[88] This study also showed that fish and moderate alcohol consumption were associated with lower risk of heart disease as well. Meats and dairy, on the other hand, were associated with a higher risk.

The American Dietetic Association stated that "appropriately planned vegetarian diets are healthful, nutritiously adequate and provide health benefits in the prevention and treatment of certain diseases."[89] In their position paper on vegetarianism, they claimed that fresh plants are good for people's health: "A considerable body of scientific data suggests positive relationships between vegetarian diet and risk reduction for several chronic degenerative diseases and conditions, including obesity, coronary artery disease, hypertension, diabetes mellitus, and some types of cancer."[90] Notably, while many of the association's members no doubt eat meat, it has never publicly stated that non-plant foods (e.g., meats) help prevent chronic disease as well.

The Case against (Red and Processed) Meats

Certain ideas about how meats are necessary for a healthy diet are simply wrong. First, people don't need meat to get complete proteins (i.e., all eight essential amino acids). People can get them by eating two plant foods together, legumes and whole grains. According to the American Dietetic Association, "[p]lant sources of protein alone can provide adequate amounts of the essential and nonessential amino adds, assuming that dietary protein sources from plants are reasonably varied and that caloric intake is sufficient to meet energy needs. Whole grains, legumes, vegetables, seeds, and nuts all contain essential and nonessential amino acids. Conscious combining of these foods within a given meal... is unnecessary."[91]

Second, people can get enough proteins from a non-meat diet. The Food and Nutrition Board of the Institute of Medicine says a person should eat roughly 0.35 grams of protein for each pound of one's body weight (or 0.8 grams of protein per kilogram) daily.[92] Because our bodies digest plant proteins differently than proteins from animals, the Vegetarian Resource Group (VRG) recommends 0.45 grams of plant-protein for each pound of weight (or about 1 gram of protein per kilogram). For a person weighing 120 pounds, that is 55 grams of protein from plants.

You can attain this level easily eating a healthy Indian diet. Legumes, grain foods, nuts, and some leafy vegetables are packed with protein. For example, a cup of garbanzo beans provides 12 grams of protein, a cup of *dal* (lentils) provides 18 grams, a slice of whole-grain bread provides 5 grams, and a handful (or 2 ounces) of almonds provides 8 grams of protein.[93] Even a cup of spinach has 5 grams of protein. A person who eats three meals a day needs about 18 grams of protein per meal. The VRG has a great table of proteins at the following URL: www.vrg.org/nutrition/protein.htm. (Their data comes from the USDA.)

Finally, people can get as many vitamins and minerals from plant foods as they can from meats, dairies, and eggs. All of this isn't to say you shouldn't eat meat, milk products, or eggs. That is your choice, but the science shows that you don't *need* to have them in order to have a balanced diet. And though meats pack the most proteins, eating too many proteins daily is bad, as it is linked to the increased risk of kidney disease and osteoporosis.[94,95]

A Wider Case against Animal-Based Foods

It is increasingly clear that red and processed meats are linked to chronic diseases. Researchers at the National Cancer Institute surveyed about 500,000 Americans aged 50 to 71 years over a period 8 years and concluded the higher the consumption of processed and red meats, the higher the risk of cancers of the lungs, esophagus, liver, colon and rectum.[96] Among the fifth of respondents who ate the most red and processed meats, their risk of developing colon cancer was 20% higher, and 16% higher for lung cancer. This wasn't due to saturated fats or proteins according to the researchers but to carcinogens like sodium nitrite in processed meats.

Health experts like Dr. Caldwell B. Esselstyn, Jr., who wrote "Prevent and Reverse Heart Disease,"[viii] and Dr. T. Colin Campbell, who wrote "The China Study," believe all foodstuffs from animals, including dairies, should be eliminated from your diet to prevent heart disease and cancers.

Let's look at why they arrived at this conclusion. When he worked in the Philippines, Dr. Campbell observed that a disproportionate number of children were developing liver cancer, which was initially

---

[viii] Caldwell B. Esselstyn, Jr.'s son, Rip Esselstyn, wrote a book titled "The Engine 2 Diet" based on similar principles.

linked to the carcinogen afla-toxin. But he discovered that there was a stronger association among the children with cancer and how much protein they ate. This observation compelled Dr. Campbell to forge a partnership between Cornell University, Oxford, and the Chinese Academy of Preventive Medicine.

This led to a 20-year study in rural China and Taiwan where Dr. Campbell found that "people who ate the most animal-based foods got the most chronic disease, [while people] who ate the most plant-based foods were the healthiest and tended to avoid chronic disease."[97] Dr. Esselstyn, who advised former U.S. President Bill Clinton on how to get into better shape, goes one step further. He tells people to not only drop animal products, but also all oils.

Working as a cardiac surgeon, Dr. Esselstyn developed the belief that fats in cooking oils led to atherosclerosis. He claimed that on his diet of only plant foods, "the average total cholesterol levels of his research group dropped from 246 to 137 mg/dL in 17 patients who followed it for five years."[98] Those 17 patients had 49 cardiac events between them before they started his diet and zero cardiac events during the five years they were on the diet.

You may benefit from reading their books and weighing the evidence. I find their conclusions compelling and agree overall with their message that a plant-based diet is the best pattern of foods for keeping people healthy. But for me, there is enough evidence to show that some fermented dairy products like *dahi* (i.e., yogurt) are beneficial. Furthermore, regarding the China Study, some peoples, like those from India and Northern Europe, tolerate lactose (the sugar in milk) better throughout their lives than other peoples, notably people from East Asia, and this general fact may confound what was observed in rural China.

Regarding an oil-free diet, there isn't enough good evidence to say that all oils are harmful. Oils have been used for cooking and dressing foods for millennia and seem to provide – certainly in the case of olive oil in the Mediterranean diet – some benefits to health. Thus, I don't see the wisdom in completely giving up dairies and oils. However, I agree with them and others that there is great wisdom in giving up most animal foods, certainly red and processed meats, from the standpoint of good health.

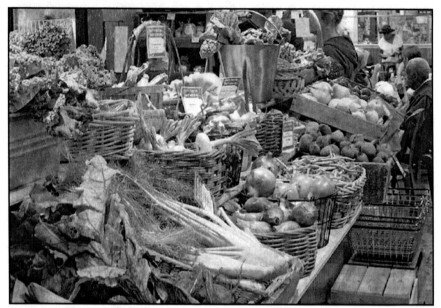

Figure 9: Plants section at a grocery store. (Photo used under Creative Commons by pwbaker.)

Other Conceptions about a Mostly Plant Diet

The American Dairy Association has done a good job persuading people that they have to drink milk to get their daily requirement of calcium. The truth is that many plants provide enough calcium. A cup of collard greens contains 400 mg of calcium. (8 ounces of milk in comparison has 300 mg of calcium.) Tempeh, a traditional Japanese food made of fermented soy, provides 200 mg per cup. A cup of cooked kale or soybean provides about 200 mg, a cup of okra or mustard greens about 150 mg, and a cup of cooked broccoli or a handful of almonds (2 ounces) about 100 mg.[99]

Generally, you need 1,000 mg of calcium daily; if you are over 50, you need 1,200 mg of calcium daily to prevent osteoporosis. In this case, supplementation with a glass of fortified orange juice (300 mg calcium) would be helpful.

Moving on, some people want to be on a low-carb diet to lose weight, or to keep it off, but vegetables and most fruits can still be eaten without affecting the goal of weight loss.[ix] This is because while they are carbohydrate-dense, vegetables, fruits, and even legumes have fiber and are made of harder to digest cabs, thereby reducing the likelihood of big glucose and insulin spikes, which is the underlying goal of low-carb diets.

Generally, simple or easy to digest carbohydrates found in refined grains, sugars, and starchy foods like potatoes should be avoided to prevent the development of chronic diseases. Meanwhile, whole grains, vegetables, fruits, and legumes contain harder to digest carbohydrates and fibers, which help people remain lean; overweight people lose body fat, keep blood sugar and insulin levels normal, and reduce the risk of developing chronic diseases. The bottom line on low-carb diets is that if you go low-carb, go low on the bad carbs, not on the good carbs found in natural, unrefined plants foods.

KINDS OF VEGETABLES AND FRUITS

I briefly describe various plant foods to clarify which vegetables and fruits are the healthiest and ought to be part of a healthy Indian diet. For this section, I owe a great debt to the works of Dr. Willett and Dr. Servan-Schreiber.

Cruciform Vegetables

Cabbage, broccoli, cauliflower, Brussels sprouts, radish, and mustard greens contain an abundance of sulforaphanes and indoles, which prevent cancer cells from becoming tumors, promote the death (apoptosis) of cancer cells, and block the process of blood vessel growth to tumors. You will get more nutrition from these vegetables if you steam or quickly stir-fry them. These cruciform vegetables also

---

[ix] Check the Harvard Glycemic Load list to figure out which fruits have a GL greater than 20 and thus should be avoided at the following URL: www.health.harvard.edu/newsweek/Glycemic_index_and_glycemic_load_for_100_foods.htm.

contain thiocyanates and nitriles, phytonutrients that may protect against some cancers.

Carotenoids-Rich Plants

Carrots, yams, sweet potatoes, squash, pumpkins, tomatoes, beets, apricots, and other vegetables that have a deep orange, red, or yellow hue are dense in carotenoids like beta-carotene (vitamin A). In a study of 22,000 American male doctors, those who ate the most beta-carotene-rich vegetables over a 12-year period had the greatest reduction in the risk of having coronary heart disease.[100] These vegetables also have lutein, phytoene, and canthaxanthin, which stimulate the immune system to attack tumor cells by encouraging Natural Killer cells to become aggressive.

Tomatoes contain lycopene, which appears to inhibit cancer cell growth. To get the most lycopene, tomatoes should be moderately cooked at low heat or by steaming, or mashed into a tomato base or salsa. The consumption of tomatoes reduced the progression of prostate cancer in a study of about 400 men, apparently due to lycopene; the consumption of fish was also shown to reduce progression, but not to the same degree as eating tomatoes.[101]

Berries, Plums, and Pomegranates

Berries like raspberries, blueberries, blackberries, cranberries, and strawberries (not actually a berry) contain an abundance of polyphenols like ellagic acid, which stimulate the liver to rid the blood of carcinogenic substances and promote self-death (apoptosis) of cancer cells. Berries also contain abundant antioxidants (e.g.,vitamin C) which reduce free radicals in the blood, and other phytonutrients shown to reduce TNF alpha and other pro-inflammatory molecules.[102] Plums, peaches, nectarines, apricots and other "stone fruits" have many of the same anti-inflammatory phytochemicals. Phytonutrients in several varieties of peaches and plums decreased the growth of human breast cancer cells in the lab setting.[103]

Pomegranate, a fruit native to India and Iran, has been used in

Ayurvedic medicine for millennia. Abundant in anti-inflammatory and antioxidant phytonutrients, pomegranate juice has shown the ability to slow the progression of prostate cancer. After a phase II clinical trial sponsored by a pomegranate marketer demonstrated this in men drinking 8 ounces of pomegranate juice every day for 2 years, the National Cancer Institute decided to fund a phase III clinical trial to determine whether pomegranate is in fact an anti-cancer food.[104]

Citrus Fruits

Oranges, tangerines, lemons, and grapefruit are rich in vitamin C, an antioxidant that appears to reduce the severity and duration of the common cold, and flavinoids, which help detoxify the body of carcinogens. Phytonutrients in the skin of citrus fruits like limonene, coumarin, and tangeritin are also believed to have anti-cancer abilities. Oranges, cultivated in India (*narangah* is Sanskrit for orange and is the root word for orange in Indo-European languages including English), contain yet other phytonutrients like pectin that seem to boost the immune system.

Garlic and other Lily Vegetables

Asparagus, chives, onions, and garlic contain a number of healthy sulfur-containing compounds. Garlic has been a medicinal herb since 3,000 B.C. Garlic paste was put into bandages used by soldiers during the world wars to prevent infections, and it has recently been shown to have anti-cancer properties.

Epidemiological studies show reduced incidences of kidney and prostate cancer among people who eat the most garlic. The sulfur compounds in these vegetables reduce the carcinogenic influence of nitrosamines, found in grilled meat and cigarette smoke, and other cancer-causing toxins. They also promote self-death (apoptosis) of several cancers.

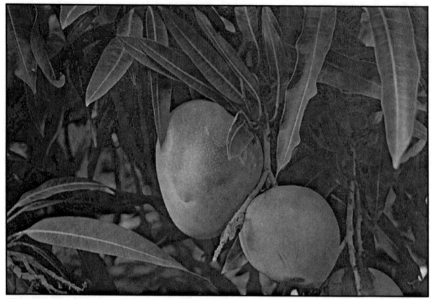

Figure 10: Mango fruit hanging on tree. (Photo used under Creative Commons from Brian Richardson.)

Mango

Mangifera indica has been cultivated in India since antiquity. Indeed, the Tamil word "maangai" became the root word for the fruit all over the world via the Portuguese. The mango is well-loved on the Subcontinent, being the national fruit of India and Pakistan. Seen in the hand of the Hindu god Lord Ganesha, its leaves are used for occasions from housewarmings to weddings, and its tangy yet sweet taste accompanies many a meal.

The pulp is one of the most phytonutrient-dense foods on the planet. It contains antioxidants in the forms of vitamin A, C, and E, several vitamin B's, carotenoids, and polyphenols. A recently discovered phytochemical named lupeol in mangoes was shown to encourage cancer cells to die, reducing the chance that they would become tumors, in mice grafted with skin cancer.[105] The mango peel contains lutein and beta-carotene, which gives them their beautiful yellow-orange color.

The Potato is Not a Part of a Healthy Diet

Native to the Americas, the potato made it to Europe via the Spaniards in the 1600s. Potatoes came to India via the Portuguese, who settled along the western coast. The potato has been popular in these regions ever since. Historians believe the potato helped ignite the population boom in Europe during the 16th and 17th centuries, and likely so in India. This is because they are calorie-dense, easy-to-digest starches, and easy to grow. During famines, the potato was a health food; it kept people alive.

But in times of plenty, where there is access to other natural foods, potatoes are *not* healthy. While they have fiber and some vitamins, they are rich in starch and thus not good on the whole, behaving like refined grains and sugars inside your body. Potatoes lead to large blood glucose and insulin surges, as their relatively high Glycemic Load tell us, which in turn encourages visceral fat growth, making people fatter. Insulin levels remain conceivably high on a diet based on potatoes, which then leads to insulin resistance, which in turn is connected to chronic diseases. Thus, potatoes are *not* a part of the healthy Indian diet.

FINAL WORD

The healthy Indian diet is mostly made up of plants for two reasons. First, plants are the basis of traditional Indian cooking, which has been abandoned thanks to the modernization of our foods. Second, there is more evidence by the day showing that plant-based diets, whether it be Indian, Mediterranean, or from another part of the world, are the healthiest.

The *National Geographic Magazine* published an essay in 2005 entitled "The Secrets of Long Life." Journalist Dan Buettner profiled people in Sardinia, Italy, Okinawa, Japan, and Loma Linda, California, claiming they were the healthiest people in the world based on how long they lived and how often without disease well into old age.[106] Buettner then wrote a book called "Blue Zones" and identified a fourth such people in Costa Rica.

I was surprised that an American group, the Loma Lindans, was considered among the healthiest in the world. From everything I had read, Americans seemed to be among the unhealthiest people in the industrialized world from the standpoint of chronic diseases. But what I discovered is that the Loma Lindans, a mostly white community connected by their Seventh-day Adventist faith, have an almost exclusively vegetarian diet.

The Seventh-day Adventists' diet has been thoroughly studied. Findings from that research are summarized by the group's dietetic association.

Since 1954 more than 250 articles have been published in scientific journals on the Seventh-day Adventist lifestyle and health. In the 1960s, Loma Linda University, in cooperation with the National Cancer Institute, began to study the health of SDAs. Later, in the 1970s and 1980s, data on the Seventh-day Adventist lifestyle was collected and analyzed under contract with the National Institutes of Health.

SDAs in general, have 50% less risk of heart disease, certain types of cancers, strokes, and diabetes. More specifically, recent data suggests that vegetarian men under 40 can expect to live more than eight years longer and women more than seven years longer than the general population. SDA vegetarian men live more than three years longer than SDA men who eat meat.

Researchers believe this added length of life and quality of health is due in particular to the consumption of whole grains, fruits and vegetables as well as the avoidance of meat, alcohol, coffee and tobacco.

Current evidence demonstrates that the more closely a person follows the lacto-ovo-vegetarian diet [that is, a diet composed of fruits, vegetables, milk, and eggs] the lower the risks of major diseases.[107]

Many months after coming across the *National Geographic* essay, I learned that parts of India may have among the lowest rate of neurodegenerative disease like Alzheimer's dementia in the world.[108] Scientists believe that if this is in fact true, it is likely due to the presence of turmeric and other spices in what people eat every day.

I often wonder: Had people eating their traditional Indian diets been able to live well into old age, historically speaking, would experts have found a Blue Zone in India? After all, the traditional Indian diet has all the elements of good health, being mostly plant-based.

Bottom Line: The healthy Indian diet is mostly plants. Plants give your body vitamins, minerals, and antioxidants, molecules that are anti-inflammatory, and other phytonutrients. Studies show that people who eat a diet rich in vegetables and fruits live longer, healthier lives.

DALS AND OTHER LEGUMES

The versatile *dal* (lentil) is a staple food in all parts of India. The dry seeds of the *Lens culinaris* plant have fed people in India, Persia, Ethiopia, and even Europe for hundreds of years, and still today, people in these regions eat lentils regularly because they taste good and are, when combined with whole grain foods, among the best sources of protein in the plant kingdom.

Soupy dishes made from *dals* are the perfect comfort food for cold days. They also make the ideal thing to go with wild rice. Try Gujarati *Daar* (page 149), which has a medley of flavors – tangy, sweet, and sour. Then there is *sambar* (page 147), which is commonly eaten in South India with *idli* and *dosa* and packs a lot of heat. You will find more legume-based recipes in Part III.

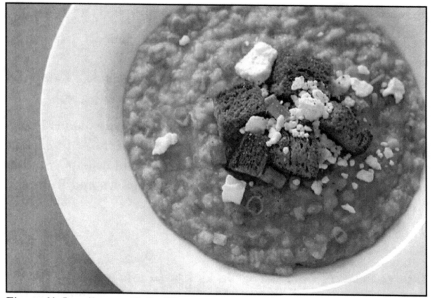

Figure 11: Lentil soup (dal). (Photo used under Creative Commons from little blue hen.)

Benefits of Legumes

Dals (lentils) are but one member of the legume family. Other legumes include various beans, peas, soybeans, chickpeas, and peanuts. What's good about legumes? First, they are protein-rich, which is important for basic sustenance and to help satisfy hunger (and thus prevent eating too much food, especially bad carbohydrates). Legumes not only provide protein, they provide fiber and nutrients.

In fact, legumes are rich in fiber. Fiber, as you recall, prevents large glucose and insulin spikes in the blood. This is why they are said to help people control their blood sugar.

Also thanks to fiber, legumes help people better control their cholesterol levels. On a related note, a diet high in soluble fiber (like a diet with lentils) is associated with a lower risk of heart disease. In a study of about 10,000 American adults, those eating at least 21 grams of fiber per day had a 10% lower risk of coronary and other cardiovascular disease compared with those who ate 5 or less grams of fiber.[109] As a reference, a half-cup (or 4 ounces) of lentils have about 6 grams of fiber.[110]

Other plentiful nutrients in legumes may explain their beneficial effects on the heart. According to the non-profit George Mateljan Foundation, there are significant amounts of folate and magnesium in legumes. Folate reduces homocysteine in the blood, a molecule believed to damages arteries and promote coronary disease. Magnesium is called "Nature's calcium channel blocker," being able to treat high blood pressure and prevent deaths from heart attacks. This is because magnesium opens up arteries, inhibits clot formation, and prevents arrhythmias.[111]

Indians have been eating a variety of lentils for generations. They include *toor dal*, the foundation of the hot South Indian *sambar;* yellow split peas; *chana dal*; *kala chana*, which is named *"desi* chickpeas" in some parts of North America; red lentils, known as *masoor dal*; *rajma* or kidney beans; and the versatile *urad dal*, used to make *dal makhani* in Punjab, *pitha* in East India, and *idli* and *dosa* in the south.[112]

Lentils aren't the only legumes in the healthy Indian diet. There are *chana* (chickpeas or garbanzo beans), for example, which are used to make a popular dish in North India called *chana masala* (as well as Mediterranean fare like falafel and hummus). Chickpeas contain molybdenum, a compound that detoxifies sulfites and are used as preservatives in many foods.

Like other legumes such as green peas, lima beans, pinto beans, and soybeans, chickpeas reduce LDL-cholesterol levels.[113] They also have a significant amount of iron and manganese, which is believed to help cells fight free radicals.[114] Clearly, *dals* and legumes are the healthiest source of proteins in the healthy Indian diet.

Bottom Line: Legumes are the main source of proteins in the healthy Indian diet. They have fiber and other nutrients that protect the heart and help control blood sugar.

SPICES

Spices – specific kinds and the extent to which they are used – make Indian culinary traditions stand apart from the other great culinary traditions of the word. India was known throughout antiquity as the land of spices, and it still is. Merchants from the Middle East and Africa sailed to the Malabar Coast for spices with the monsoon winds, and Marco Polo sought a quicker, safer route to India's spices as the demand increased in Europe.

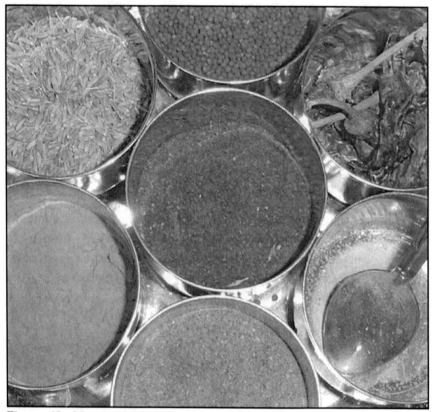

Figure 12: Masala dabi (spice collection). (Photo used under Creative Commons from madpai.)

Indians use spices in cooking for more than just taste. They are also seen as being medicinal. Ayurvedic practices coalescing around 1500 B.C. influenced the use of spices in everyday food. In the following pages, I will describe the Indian spices that have the most scientific support for playing a role in preventing inflammation and fighting chronic disease.

Spices are what give Indian dishes their distinctive flavors. Some you may be familiar with, like cinnamon with its spicy and sweet aroma. Ginger and garlic aren't technically spices but are used to spice up dishes. Turmeric is uniquely Indian, and though it is bitter, people add a dash of this for its deep yellow-orange color and medicinal qualities. It is useful to think of spices as mixes and not as individual ingredients because that is how they are used in Indian cooking. Plus, there is synergy among the individual spices found in curry powder (page 182) and *garam masala* (page 180) that give them their remarkable influence on health.

Turmeric

Turmeric (*haldi* in Hindi), historically called "Indian saffron" outside the Subcontinent because of its deep yellow-orange color, is an essential part of healthy Indian diets. This is because of its bioactive compound, one that gives turmeric its characteristic color and powerful anti-inflammatory power: curcumin.

The turmeric plant (*Curcuma longa*) is in the ginger or *Zingiberaceae* family and native to tropical South India. The rhizomes (i.e., roots) are cultivated, boiled, dried, and finally ground to make the powder, which has a slightly peppery, bitter taste and mustard-like scent. It is also used for medicinal purposes based on Ayurvedic tradition.

Dr. Bharat Aggarwal, an M. D. Anderson Cancer Center researcher, has elucidated much of what is known about curcumin's ability to fight cancer. According to his website, curcumin is only ½ of a gram for every 25 grams of turmeric powder.[115] Outside of food, Dr. Aggarwal believes purified curcumin may be helpful if given concurrently with chemotherapy and radiotherapy in certain cancer patients because of its anti-inflammatory abilities and lack of side effects.

Several studies show that curcumin seems to shrink tumors in animals. A 2010 study from UCLA demonstrated that the growth of head-and-neck tumors grafted on mice was better suppressed in mice treated with both curcumin and conventional chemotherapy compared with mice treated with chemotherapy alone.[116] Dr. Aggarwal's team showed that 500 mg/kg of curcumin suppressed the actions of NF-kappa B, which promotes cancer cells to live forever and grow, to such extent that tumors from various cancers grafted onto mice actually shrunk.[117] That curcumin seems to suppress the actions of NF-kappa B may explain why it seems to prevent and treat cancer in mice.

A 1997 New England Journal of Medicine review recognized that NF-kappa B was the central transcription factor for the development of diseases caused by inflammation.[118] In 2007, a review in Clinical Oncology recognized the central role that NF-kappa B plays in the formation of cancer in humans.[119]

This evidence suggests that by inhibiting NF-kappa B, turmeric powder may prevent the formation of cancer when it is simply a few isolated cancer cells and before they coalesce into a tumor. Some health experts also believe that turmeric powder helps prevent Alzheimer's disease, although this association is based on the observation that people in rural India have low rates of neurodegenerative disease, which has not been more extensively studied.[120]

That said, Alzheimer's disease is beginning to be seen as an inflammatory disease. One body of evidence has shown that the regular use of NSAIDs like aspirin, which reduce general inflammation, are associated with lower rates of Alzheimer's disease.[121] Like NSAIDs, curcumin is believed to lower inflammation by reducing leukotrienes, prostaglandins, and thromboxanes levels. A 2005 review cited studies that showed curcumin was associated with lower levels of molecular oxidation by free radicals (i.e., it behaved as an antioxidant) and beta-amyloid, the protein most intimately linked to Alzheimer's disease.[122]

Moving on, curcumin seems to improve cholesterol in the blood. In one study, 500 mg of curcumin was given to 10 healthy people daily for 7 days. HDL-cholesterol increased by about 30%, while total cholesterol decreased by about 10% – a good outcome.[123] Furthermore, the amount of oxidized fat molecules in the blood fell after the 7 days on curcumin by about 30% – also a good thing. I don't want to draw strong conclusions from this one small study, but considering the central role that inflammation plays in atherosclerosis, turmeric powder can likely protect the heart from coronary disease.

Black Peppercorn

Most people have black pepper after the dried peppercorn fruit of the *Piper nigrum* plant is crushed. Black pepper is known in Ayurvedic tradition to improve digestion. As evidence, peppercorn's bioactive compound piperine improved the absorption of curcumin in people's blood by 2,000% (though this was purified piperine in a high-dose pill, not peppercorn).[124] Piperine has seems to reduce pain at a molecular level.[125]

Bottom Line: The critical spice in the healthy Indian diet is turmeric powder, which contains curcumin, an anti-inflammatory antioxidant. To improve the absorption of curcumin, add ground black peppercorn.

Garlic

People have been eating garlic cloves and using them for medicinal purposes for hundreds of years. Most studies on garlic have been carried out on extract or powder from the cloves. A 2006 *Journal of Nutrition* review shows that garlic extract and powder seem to reduce total cholesterol in people with high levels, lower blood pressure, and decrease platelet aggregation, which could help prevent the kind of clot that causes both heart attacks and strokes.[126] In the lab setting, garlic has been shown to reduce inflammation.

Ginger

The rhizome (i.e., root) of the *Zingibier officianale* plant seems to reduce inflammation in some studies, which may explain why it is used traditionally for joint pain. In about 250 people with osteoarthritis of the knee, the subjects taking ginger extract had better pain relief compared with those who took a placebo.[127] Ginger extract reduces the production of prostaglandins and TNF-alpha, both proinflammation molecules, and thus behaves like ibuprofen and similar NSAIDs.[128] Ginger also demonstrated the ability to reduce the formation of new cancer cells in mice grafted with skin cancer.

Red Chili Pepper

The most popular red chili pepper is the cayenne pepper, which is especially high in the antioxidant vitamin A. (The *Capsicum* plants are not related to the plants that produce peppercorn, from which black pepper is made.) The bioactive molecule capsaicin seems to reduce pain at a molecular level. In fact, a relatively new medication for osteoarthritic joints and painful inflammatory skin disease like psoriasis is a topical cream of capsaicin. In addition to having anti-inflammatory qualities, eating red chili pepper may reduce your risk of heart disease.

Oxidation of lipoproteins (i.e., LDL) in 27 patients eating a cayenne pepper blend daily for 4 weeks was lower compared with a matched group on a similar diet but without the pepper.[129] Many heart experts claim that oxidized lipoproteins are the trigger for clinically significant coronary disease. Capsaicin seems to also inhibit the activation of NF-kappa B, the cancer promoting inflammatory molecule, in mice grafted with prostate cancer. The authors postulated that capsaicin may also slow the progression of prostate cancer disease in men.[130]

Cinnamon

Cinnamon powder, acquired from the bark of the *Cinnamomum* tree, appears helpful in diabetics. Ground cinnamon, once digested, seems to help cells get the insulin signal, which they were otherwise ignoring. A 2003 study showed that people with diabetes who had 1 gram of ground cinnamon (in a capsule) for 40 straight days had substantially lower fasting blood sugar, LDL-cholesterol, and triglyceride levels 20 days afterwards when compared with a matched group of diabetics who had a placebo capsule.[131]

However, not all studies showed this effect. Two studies using the same amount of ground cinnamon, one of type 1 diabetic teenagers (type 1 is not associated with obesity) and the other of postmenopausal type 2 diabetic women, did not show better or worse effects on blood glucose or lipids.[132,133] Nonetheless, there is evidence that in some diabetics, ground cinnamon improves their blood glucose, cholesterol, and triglycerides, and without side effects.

Other Spices and Synergy

The spices I have described above are ones where the scientific evidence is somewhat compelling. But they aren't the only spices in the healthy Indian diet. Coriander seeds (*dhania*), like the leaves, contain antioxidants, but their effects have not been studied in people. They do lower blood glucose, cholesterol, and triglyceride levels in animals, and have historically been used for diabetes treatment in India.[134,135] Cumin (*jeera*) promotes proper digestion according to the Ayurvedic tradition, and eating cumin did increase digestive enzymes levels in a limited study.[136] It was also shown to lower the ability of platelets to form clots.[137]

There isn't as much evidence to support the health claims of other spices in Indian diets, like cardamom (*elaichi*), mustard seeds (*rai*) and asafetida (*heeng*), but that doesn't mean you should avoid them. In general, spices contain antioxidant and anti-inflammatory abilities as well as minerals and vitamins, much of which modern science has yet to study. More important is that a particular spice is likely able to provide you more benefit when other spices are present.

This potential synergy is little studied by scientists today. After all, there isn't much money to be made by studying spices, as they are food commodities that most people will use for taste regardless of what the science says. But recall the evidence showing how more curcumin (in turmeric) is absorbed in people's blood when piperine (in black peppercorn) was also present in the digestive tract. Hopefully, these studies will be done more often, allowing us to see the bigger picture. Until then, what we have to go by mostly in terms of using a variety of spices together for the maximal benefit is the recognition by Ayurvedic traditions, honed by experiments over millennia, that there were synergies between spices.

Curry Powder and Garam Masala

Here I describe two general combinations of Indian spices influenced by the Ayurvedic tradition of mixing individual components that had synergistic relationships so that the whole is greater than the sum of the parts.

Curry powder, a Western concoction, is a common combination for South Indian dishes today. (The word curry comes from the Tamil word *kari.*) Most commercial curry powders contain coriander, turmeric, cumin, fenugreek, and dried ginger. The manufacturer, or you if you make your own curry powder, may add dried garlic, asafoetida, fennel seed, caraway, cinnamon, clove, mustard seed, green cardamom, black cardamom, mace, nutmeg, long pepper, black pepper, and red chili pepper.

Garam masala is more commonly used in North Indian dishes. In general, *garam masala* (meaning hot spices in Hindi) contain ground cinnamon, cloves, cardamom, nutmeg, and black peppercorn. Similar to curry powder, the spices I listed above or others can be added to suit your taste.

Bottom Line: Spices of all kinds are an essential component of the healthy Indian diet. There is synergy between spices that makes the whole greater than the sum of its parts, so use them in traditional mixes.

DAHI AND OTHER FERMENTED DAIRIES

Dahi (yogurts), *raita*, *lassi*, curds, butter and *ghee* have always been commonly eaten in India. This may be why Hindus have held cows in high esteem, having relied on them for basic sustenance since ancient times. And their beneficial effects on the body are likely why these fermented dairies are an essential component of the healthy Indian diet.

Dahi is a versatile accompaniment to many dishes in all corners of India because it is easy to make (you only need milk and a little bit of "starter *dahi*," check out page 168) and cools off the intense heat generated when you ingest spices. It is also the foundation for the refreshingly cool, creamy Punjabi drink popular at Indian restaurants, *lassi* (page 172). You can discover more recipes for fermented dairies in Part III.

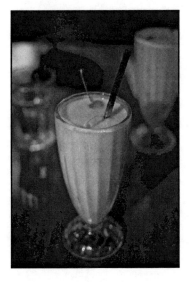

Figure 13: Lassi made from *dahi* (yogurt). (Photo used under Creative Commons from Joey)

Lower Colon Cancer Risk

Your intestines contain hundreds of bacteria, some good and some bad. Diarrhea and bleeding are often the result of bad bacteria taking over the colon, but good bacteria like *Lactobacillus acidophilus*, when they become dominant, ease bowel movements and thereby reduce the time your body is exposed to carcinogenic substances. These bacteria, along with *Lactococcus* species, are common in Indian dairies like *dahi*.[138]

Some dairies seem to prevent colon cancer. A 2001 *American Journal of Clinical Nutrition* review stated that bacteria found in probiotics like *dahi* limited the development of cancerous cells in the colon.[139] In a study of almost 61,000 Swedish women, those who ate high-fat dairy products, which included whole milk, cultured milk, cheese, cream, sour cream, and butter, at least 4 times daily had a 41% lower risk of developing colon cancer than those who did not.[140]

The authors believed that conjugated linoleic acid (CLA), a fatty acid in dairy products, was responsible for this reduced risk. Dairies' impact on the immune system may also inhibit colon cancer. In women at least, eating a lot of fermented dairies made certain immune cells, T and Natural Killer cells, more aggressive against abnormal (e.g., cancer) cells.[141,142]

Reduction of Visceral Body Fat and Insulin Resistance

Fermented dairies are high in proteins and calcium. Calcium is important for keeping bones strong and for keeping muscles, including the heart, functioning normally. Proper calcium levels in the blood may also help with weight loss.

Dr. Michael Zimmel, a University of Tennessee researcher, has found that eating foods rich in calcium like *dahi* helps the body lose excess body fat. In one of his studies, weight loss in 16 patients on 400-500 mg of daily calcium was compared with 18 patients on 1,100 mg of daily calcium from being on a yogurt diet. Both groups adhered to the same exercise and calorie regimen.

After 12 weeks, the higher-calcium group lost more abdominal fat (i.e., visceral fat).[143] The authors said that "isocaloric substitution of yogurt for other foods significantly augments fat loss and reduces central adiposity during energy restriction." Observational studies found an association between high consumption of dairies and lower visceral body fat in different people.[144,145]

This may explain why higher-calcium diets prevent overweight people from developing insulin resistance (which often leads to diabetes and heart disease). In one such demonstration among 3,100 young American adults, those who were overweight and said they ate at least 35 servings of dairies each week (foods made of some milk, like sour cream dip, counted as a dairy in this study) had a 72% lower risk of developing signs of insulin resistance compared with those who were overweight and ate less than 10 servings of dairies per week.[146]

Experts believe that as calcium enters fat cells, it induces the release of free fatty acids and triglycerides into the blood. The body's other cells use these fat molecules for fuel. Meanwhile, visceral fat tissue stops growing or even shrinks.[147] This is the likely explanation why eating fermented dairies like *dahi* seems to help with weight loss.

Bottom Line: Fermented dairies like *dahi*, *raita*, and *lassi* are a part of the healthy Indian diet. They help the colon stay healthy, introduce good bacteria into the body, and seem to help people lose excess body fat.

PICKLES AND CHUTNEYS

Indians love *achar* (a variety of pickled plant foods in Hindi) and other pickled foods. The tradition of pickling plant foods has been around since ancient times, when it was the only reliable way to preserve foods. Like fermented dairies and *kimchi*, a fermented cabbage dish from Korea, Indian pickles are made by anaerobic bacteria.

They are mostly made by letting fruit or vegetables ferment in a bottle of vinegar. Sometimes, oils, spices, and salt are added. Indian pickles are typically made from mango, lime, Indian gooseberry, bitter melon, chili pepper, turmeric root, ginger, and garlic. Chutneys are a popular form of pickled products (although some chutneys are pastes rather than pickles) that add a tangy flavor to dishes.

Lactobacillus is the dominant bacteria in pickles. They make lactic acid during fermentation, giving pickles a sour taste to balance the natural sweetness of the fruit. In the colon, *Lactobacillus* helps keep bacteria that promote inflammation at bay. The more fermented foods you eat, the more likely it is that the good anaerobic bacteria will become the dominant bacteria in your colon. They benefit the body by reducing the effects of bad bacteria and by producing vitamins and short-chain fatty acids.

You will find Indian pickles and chutneys taste nothing like what you might consider to be a pickle (e.g., pickled cucumber). They range from a fresh and light dipping sauce (see coriander *chutney* on page 174) to a thick, sweet-and-sour dressing with some crunch (see mango pickle on page 178).

Bottom Line: Pickles and chutneys made by fermenting are a regular condiment in the healthy Indian diet.

BROWN RICE AND WHOLE GRAINS

Rice and leavened grains like *naans* are commonly eaten all over India. Traditionally, mostly whole grain foods were eaten, but since the food supply was modernized beginning in the early 1900s, refined grain products have become more abundant in India like white rice, a refined product of brown rice, and finely-ground grains like *maida* (all-purpose flour or plain flour).

However, if you go back to eating grains the way they were traditionally eaten, you will find they taste more like the earth from which they came. Brown rice, for example, is nuttier and chewier than white rice, which has a simpler starchy flavor. No matter what is mixed into a *paratha*, the soft heartiness of the *atta* (whole wheat flour) dominates its taste. (Find recipes for spinach and *methi paratha* on page 164.) Heart-healthy oats add a nuttiness to *dosa*, a crepe-like food popular in the south (see the recipe on page 156).

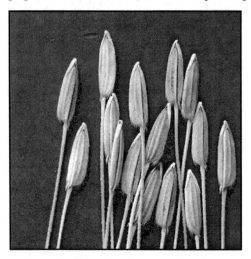

Figure 14: Wild rice grains. (Photo used under Creative Commons from International Rice Research Institute Images.)

White and Brown Rice

Rice is a staple in India. The grains of the *Oryza sativa* plant is what we call rice. In nature, rice grains are brown in color and made of two parts, the kernel and the endosperm. The kernel is itself made of two parts, the germ and the bran. Most vitamins, minerals and fatty acids are in the germ. Meanwhile, the bran, which is the outer part of the kernel, contains most of the fiber, therefore, most of the nutrition is in the kernel.

Brown rice is *lightly* milled rice that contains most of the kernels. White rice on the other hand is the end product after *heavy* milling, leaving barely any kernels (germ and bran). What's left is the endosperm, which is mostly starch. And white rice has become very common, along with other refined grains, in modern diets.

The George Mateljan Foundation claims that "complete milling and polishing that converts brown rice into white rice destroys [at least 67% of the B vitamins, including thiamine, found in brown rice], half of the manganese, half of the phosphorus, 60% of the iron, and all of the dietary fiber and essential fatty acids." Therefore, white rice is nutritiously poor.

White rice is also dense in bad carbohydrates that create problems for the glucose/insulin feedback system. The starchy endosperm has a longer shelf life without the kernel, and thus manufacturers and grocery stores prefer to market white rice because of this extended shelf life. People everywhere also prefer white rice as it takes less time to cook and tastes better to modern palettes.

However, brown rice, being a whole grain food, has much more nutritional value and fiber, which helps keep glucose and insulin levels stable, than white rice. The science increasingly shows that brown rice is good for you and that white rice is bad. The best evidence comes from a 2010 study looking at more than 197,000 people.

Two important associations emerged. First, people who ate 5 or more servings of white rice each week increased their risk of developing type 2 diabetes by 17% compared with people who ate no rice.[148] Second, people who ate a serving of brown rice at least 2 times each week *reduced* their risk of developing type 2 diabetes by 11% compared with people who ate no rice. This is worth repeating: the regular consumption of white rice increased people's risk of developing diabetes, while the regular consumption of brown rice actually decreased that risk.

Whole Grains

Brown rice is just one part of the whole grains story, all of which contain the nutrient-rich germ, fiber-rich bran, and starch-rich endosperm. In contrast, refined grains are made of mostly one of those things, the starch-rich endosperm. This is why I wrote earlier that refined grains are not only nutrition poor, but they are harmful. The science is clear that eating whole grains in general (e.g., wild rice, oats, corn, barley, whole wheat and grain breads, whole wheat pasta, millet, and quinoa) is good for you.

A 2007 review found that eating 2 servings of whole grains every day substantially reduced the risk of developing type 2 diabetes (similar to what was seen in another review where people ate brown rice).[149] This finding coincides with our understanding that whole grains, largely because of their fiber, don't cause large surges in blood glucose and insulin levels compared with refined grains. Furthermore, the regular consumption of whole grains is heart healthy. Below is a quote from the American Heart Association's premier journal.

> Dietary patterns that are high in whole-grain products and fiber have been associated with increased diet quality and decreased risk of [heart disease]. Soluble or viscous fibers (notably ß-glucan and pectin) modestly reduce LDL cholesterol levels beyond those achieved by a diet low in saturated and trans fatty acids and cholesterol alone. Insoluble fiber has been associated with decreased [heart disease] risk and slower progression of [heart disease] in high-risk individuals. Dietary fiber may promote satiety by slowing gastric emptying, leading to an overall decrease in calorie intake. Soluble fiber may increase short-chain fatty acid synthesis, thereby reducing endogenous cholesterol production. The AHA recommends that at least half of grain intake come from whole grains.[150]

In addition to helping people prevent heart disease and diabetes, whole grains help people control their weight. A study following about 27,000 middle-aged and elderly men showed that the men in general gained weight over an eight-year period, but those consuming lots of whole grains saw a smaller gain in weight.[151] The men who added bran (the fiber-rich component of grains) to their diets saw an even smaller gain in weight. (Incidentally, men eating fiber-rich cereal and fruit also had lower weight gain.)

A study of about 292,000 men and 198,000 middle-aged and elderly women followed over 10 years showed that regular consumption of whole grains was associated with a modest reduction in the risk of colon cancer.[152] As I explained earlier, fiber doesn't seem to reduce the risk of colon cancer, so perhaps vitamins, minerals or other phytonutrients in the germ and bran explain this finding. These studies show that whole grains help people lower the risk of diabetes, coronary heart disease, and colon cancer, as well as insulin resistance and bad cholesterol levels.

Traditionally speaking, Indians ate coarsely ground grains like *atta* (stone-ground wheat), brown rice, barley, rye, maize, millet, and sorghum.[153] But Indians in modern times eat more *maida* (finely ground refined wheat), white rice, and other finely ground grains. The healthy Indian diet harks back to an era before food was heavily refined.

If you want to use whole grain flours, look for flours with the word "meal," as in oatmeal or cornmeal.[x] If you like how the refined stuff tastes when you bake something but want to eat healthier, mix some coarser-grain meal into the flour.

Bottom Line: Whole grains help reduce the risk of diabetes, heart disease, and colon cancer, and are thus a part of the healthy Indian diet. White rice increases your risk of diabetes, and switching to brown rice would greatly benefit your health. When looking for whole grain flours for baking, find coarsely ground or stone-milled grains that are called "wholemeal."

---

[x] In the U.S., the FDA doesn't allow terms like "whole wheat," "whole grain" or "wholemeal" unless the product is truly whole grain or stone-ground, thus containing lots of germ and bran. However, a product can be labeled as such if greater than 50% of its contents are whole grain by weight.

COOKING OILS AND GHEE

People use cooking oils from plant sources and other fatty foods like *ghee* or butter for cooking and dressing foods. These foods are the main source of dietary fats in your diet. In this section, I write about how to use them properly, as in which ones to cook with and which ones to dress foods with, in the healthy Indian diet.

Ghee

Ghee (clarified butter) is popular in India for cooking and even religious ceremonies. It is made by melting butter over low heat until most of the water has evaporated, leaving a protein-rich layer at the bottom and a fat-rich layer, the *ghee*, on top. While *ghee* is full of saturated fats, eating it in moderation will not significantly increase your risk of coronary heart disease according to the latest science.

For example, a 2005 study in young, healthy people was done to see how *ghee* affected cholesterol levels. Thirty subjects got 10% of their daily calories from *ghee*, while 33 subjects on a similar diet ate no *ghee* at all. After 8 weeks, the cholesterol levels between the groups were not significantly differently, suggesting that *ghee* in moderation doesn't worsen cholesterol.[154]

Some fats in *ghee* are good. A quarter are medium and short-chain saturated fats, which benefit the body. But *ghee* is also rich in long-chain saturated fats, many of which are bad. Thus, *ghee* should be used moderately. According to the George Mateljan Foundation, which cited the 2005 study, eating 20 grams (i.e., 2 tablespoons) of *ghee* a day should not affect your cholesterol levels.[155]

That amount is ideal for use in cooking. Because *ghee* has a relatively high smoke-point temperature (about 485°F, whereas most cooking occurs around 400°F), it is unlikely to get unstable and release free radicals into your food like many vegetable oils might. *Ghee* can also be used to dress food, as people like to do on their *roti* and *biryani*, but again, do so in moderation.

Coconut Oil

Coconut oil is historically used in South Indian cooking. Being largely medium-chain saturated fats (i.e., MCT or MCFA in the literature), coconut oil tends not to break down and make free radicals in typical cooking heat (around 400°F), unlike many vegetable oils. The saturated fats in coconut oil are used to make hospital baby formulas and sports drinks today because they are used quickly for fuel and not stored; coconut oil has been used in these products in the past.[156,157]

Nutrition experts like Dr. Andrew Weil may not endorse recent claims about coconut products (e.g., coconut milk is the healthiest beverage), but he admits to cooking with coconut oil as it tastes good and is unlikely to promote disease.[158] A 1981 study of Tokelau Islanders near New Zealand showed that coconut oil may actually protect the health of your heart. In islanders who moved to New Zealand and adopted a Modern diet, about 40% of their daily calories came from fats. In contrast, islanders who stayed on the islands and ate their traditional diet got about 60% of their daily calories from fats, and most of that from coconut oil. The study found that the islanders who ate more dietary fats and much more coconut oil had *better* cholesterol levels.[159] Dr. Ian Prior led the Tokelau Island study and wrote, "Vascular disease is uncommon in both populations and there is no evidence of the high saturated fat intake [from coconut oil has] a harmful effect…"[160]

Supporting his claim, evidence shows that lauric acid, the most common fat in coconut oil, increases HDL-C levels more than it increases LDL-C levels – a good outcome.[161] Dr. George Blackburn, a Harvard physician, was quoted at a 1988 U.S. Congressional hearing as saying, "Coconut oil has a neutral effect on blood cholesterol, even in situations where coconut oil is the sole source of fat."[162] Based on newer science, using coconut oil every day in moderate amounts is not likely to increase your risk of developing coronary heart disease.

Canola Oil

Canola oil is used in the developed world for cooking. It comes from a strain of the rape plant that contains little erucic acid, a potentially harmful fat. But there is no compelling evidence that canola oil is in fact harmful. With a smoking point temperature above 450°F, it tends not to break down and produce free radicals from cooking heat. Furthermore, canola oil is high in monounsaturated fats, including omega-3 fatty acids.

Said University of Pittsburgh professor Dr. Robert L. Wolke, "[Canola oil] is valued for its fatty acid profile, which is 59 percent monounsaturated, 30 percent polyunsaturated and 7 percent saturated. This compares favorably with Health Champ olive oil's profile: 74 percent monounsaturated, 8 percent polyunsaturated and 14 percent saturated."[163] Because of its good fat profile and high smoke-point temperature, canola oil is ideal for cooking.

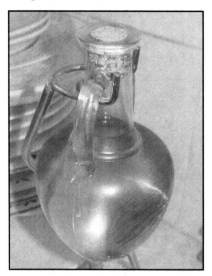

Figure 15: Bottle of olive oil. (Photo used under Creative Commons from Smabs Sputzer.)

Olive Oil

The Mediterranean diet is based on extra-virgin olive oil. Olive oil is good because it is low in saturated fat and high in monounsaturated fat, which makes up 75% of the fats in the oil. A study of about 850 Greeks with and about 1,000 Greeks without heart disease found that the exclusive use of olive oil decreased the risk of suffering a heart attack by about 50%.[164]

Eating olive oil likely reduces the risk of hypertension. A 2004 Greek study of 20,000 people without high blood pressure found that olive oil alone was responsible for keeping their blood pressures normal.[165]

However, olive oil should be had in food as a dressing for you to get its health benefits. People mistakenly use olive oil for cooking. At 350°F to 400°F, most commercially available olive oils have relatively low smoke-point temperatures. This means that many olive oils will break down under cooking heat (which is around 400°F), thus releasing free radicals. Furthermore, the excessive heat will destroy most phytonutrients like phenols and antioxidants that are believed to give extra-virgin olive oil its power.

Other Vegetable Oils

Many vegetable oils are used for cooking. Mustard oil, which has a sinus-irritating aroma, is popular in Bengal and other parts of East India. Some commercially available mustard oil has other vegetable oils like safflower oil blended in. Mustard oil was once considered bad based on rat studies without accounting for the fact that rats lack enzymes to break down mustard oil, unlike people. Mustard oil has been proven safe in people.[166]

Researchers at Harvard, All India Institute of Medical Science (AIIMS) in New Delhi, and St. John's Medical College in Bangalore looked at 350 people with and 700 people without coronary heart disease and found that people using mustard oil for cooking had a lower risk of coronary heart disease than those using sunflower oil.[167] A reasonable conclusion is that mustard oil was better for heart health than sunflower oil because of its higher monounsaturated fat level.

Corn oil is a popular cooking oil among Indian people living in the U.S. Commercially available refined corn oil has a smoke-point temperature of 450°F, which makes it suitable for cooking. Lately, corn oil has been deemed bad because of its high omega-6 fatty acid levels relative to omega-3 fatty acid, which some researchers believe promotes inflammation. But the AHA's science advisory panel found that a *small* amount of omega-6 fatty acid-rich oils like corn oil can actually lower the risk of coronary heart disease.[168] This finding underscores the importance in terms of health of eating small amounts (i.e., a few tablespoons at most) of oils.

(Partially) Hydrogenated Oils – The Worst Food

Partially hydrogenated oils are made after hydrogen atoms are added in the factory setting to the carbon backbone of an oil molecule. This refining process creates *trans* double bonds, which make oils solid at room temperature and give them longer shelf lives. Trans fats have thus become the favored kind of fat by the food and restaurant industries. But as you likely know, trans fats are probably the worst food for you. They lead to a greater risk of coronary heart disease than any other food.[169] The science here is not controversial, unlike with saturated fats. Whereas some experts tell us a moderate amount of saturated fats will do no harm, and others advocate no saturated fats, no expert I have come across says we should ever put trans fats into our bodies.

Harvard researchers looking at the diets of 240 patients who had suffered a heart attack wrote, "[Our] data support the hypothesis that intake of partially hydrogenated vegetable oils may contribute to the risk of myocardial infarction."[170] So if you have a bottle of oil at home labeled with the word "hydrogenated" or "partially hydrogenated," you shouldn't use it anymore if you can help it.

Bottom Line: Coconut oil and *ghee* are part of the healthy Indian diet in moderation (about 2 tablespoons per day). They are also ideal for cooking, as is canola oil. Olive oil should be used to dress food, not for cooking, to get its full benefits.

TREE NUTS

Disclaimer: If you are or believe you may be allergic to nuts, avoid nuts altogether. Speak with your physician if you have concerns about a nut allergy.

Nuts are heart healthy. While nuts are eaten uncooked as a dry snack, there is one dish I want to highlight where a nut is broken into small pieces and actually cooked with other ingredients: *Shahi paneer*, a curried dish made of a rich and creamy cashew-based sauce (see page 126).

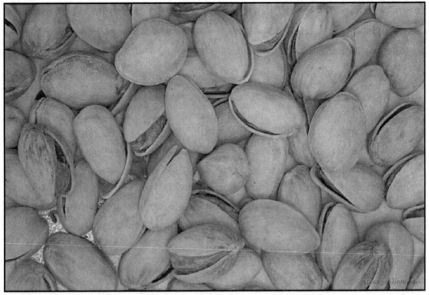

Figure 16: Pistachios. (Photo used under Creative Commons from Casey Fleser.)

Nuts are Heart-Healthy

What food increases HDL-cholesterol (i.e., the good one) while lowering LDL-cholesterol? The answer is tree nuts. In a review of almost 600 people, some with high cholesterol not taking anti-cholesterol medication, eating almost 80 grams of nuts led to a significant drop in LDL and total cholesterol levels along with an increase in HDL-cholesterol – all of which is good.[171] The reduction in LDL-cholesterol was more pronounced in those who had bad cholesterol levels to begin with.

Eating tree nuts not only improves cholesterol levels, it actually reduces the risk of coronary heart disease. Recall the Seventh-day Adventists I mentioned when discussing a plant-based diet. A study of 31,200 Adventists who ate nuts at least 4 times a week showed an almost 50% decrease in the risk of fatal heart attacks compared with those who ate nuts less than once per week.[172] This conclusion has also been reached in larger studies.

A study of 86,000 women showed that frequent consumption of nuts (5 ounces per week) decreased the risk of both fatal and non-fatal heart attacks by 35%.[173] The authors of a 2008 *Journal of Nutrition* review on nuts and heart health concluded that there must be more to the story than just good fats.

> Thus, in addition to a favorable fatty acid profile, nuts and peanuts contain other bioactive compounds that explain their multiple cardiovascular benefits. Other macronutrients include plant protein and fiber; micronutrients including potassium, calcium, magnesium, and tocopherols; and phytochemicals such as phytosterols, phenolic compounds, resveratrol, and arginine. Nuts and peanuts are food sources that are a composite of numerous cardioprotective nutrients and if routinely incorporated in a healthy diet, population risk of CHD would therefore be expected to decrease markedly.[174]

Phytonutrients in nuts probably act as antioxidants that reduce inflammation, just as they do in other plant foods. And reducing inflammation translates to a lower risk of a plaque formation in the coronary arteries.

Omega-3 fatty acid is a particularly good fat in nuts which reduces inflammation, and it is believed to relieve some autoimmune diseases and improve heart health.[175,176,177] The best nuts for omega-3 fatty acids are walnuts.[178] Nonetheless, plenty of nuts have omega-3 fatty acids and other helpful nutrients, not to mention proteins that the body needs.

Bottom Line: Tree nuts are a perfect snack in a healthy Indian diet. They help lower your risk of developing heart disease.

MODERN ELEMENTS THAT DON'T BELONG

Most of this book is devoted to what the healthy Indian diet actually *is*, but I can't fully describe the traditional Indian pattern of foods without also defining what does *not* belong. Briefly then, I will mention the stuff that makes a Modern diet, Indian or otherwise, bad for you. If you already eat plenty of Indian dishes but want to make them healthier, the easiest way to do so is to cut down on these foods.

Indian Snack Food and Refined Grains

Indian snack foods are most often fried refined grain foods made to taste savory, spicy, salty, or sweet. So in addition to refined grains, these packaged foods are full of sugar (sometimes called corn syrup or fructose) and salt (or sodium). As you may have learned many pages ago, eating easily digestible carbohydrates found in refined grains and sugar lead to large surges in blood sugar and the hormone insulin, which causes you to get fatter. Eating this stuff on a regular basis will cause you to develop insulin resistance, which is just a step or two away from diabetes and coronary heart disease.

Sugar

The simple carbs found in table sugar, high fructose corn syrup (HFCS), and other forms of sugar are easily digestible. This means they quickly go from your intestines and into your blood, flooding it with glucose and fructose. You now know that increased glucose levels lead to increased insulin levels, and that chronically elevated insulin levels lead to insulin resistance, which often leads to heart disease and diabetes.

You don't need to cut out all sugars. Reduce the artificial sugars as much as possible, but you can't avoid all sugars. You will get sugars in

113

their natural forms in some elements of the healthy Indian diet, notably fruits, but they also contain fiber, which lessens the impact sugar has on your insulin levels, and beneficial phytonutrients (e.g., vitamins, antioxidants, and anti-inflammatories) missing in table sugar and foods made with them (e.g., cookies and cakes).

There is a school of thought that advocates we should eat a little bit of table sugar with every meal. This is because we crave sugar (thanks to how our ancestors evolved in an environment where it was hard to find food), and that we will feel hungry or unsatisfied if we don't get it. Dr. Rob Thompson advocated having a teaspoon of sugar with each meal in his book on the glycemic diet.

This is because eating a little sugar like this reduces your craving for carb-dense foods like rice. Plus, a teaspoon of table sugar has a relatively low impact on your insulin levels compared with other foods. Here is an illustration of the logic behind this strategy: A teaspoon of table sugar has a Glycemic Load of 28 compared with 100 for a slice of white bread and 283 for a cup of white rice.[179]

Salt

I haven't discussed salt much because it doesn't seem to influence your glucose/insulin feedback system or inflammation levels. However, it does lead to hypertension (i.e., high blood pressure), which is the primary risk factor for strokes. It is also a risk factor for atherosclerosis and heart attacks.

The food that increases blood pressure the most seems to be table salt (i.e., sodium chloride). But it is unclear how much salt actually matters. The DASH study attempted to find out and made two discoveries related to salt. First, reducing how much salt the subjects ate from high to intermediate to low reduced blood pressure modestly, or a couple of "points" of mmHg.[180] Second, people eating the control diet (i.e., a Modern diet) plus a high amount of sodium had much higher systolic blood pressures, about 8 mmHg more in people with normal pressure, and about 12 mmHg higher in people with hypertension compared with people on the DASH diet (which emphasized fruits, vegetables, and low-fat dairy products) plus a low amount of sodium.

While these blood pressure reductions appear modest, they have a large impact on people's vulnerability to strokes and heart attacks. Therefore, it is worth cutting back on salt, even though salt is common to many Indian dishes and often unavoidable. Similar to sugar, your goal should be to eat as little salt as possible. A useful strategy is to replace salt with other spices if you want more flavor in what you eat.

Bottom Line: Cut down on pre-packaged snacks, as they mostly contain refined grains. The healthy Indian diet also contains low amounts of salt and sugar.

3 MYTHS ABOUT THE INDIAN DIET

I hear Indian uncles and aunties say these things all the time. If I don't dispel them now, people will continue holding on to these misconceptions.

1. "*Ghee* and coconut oil are bad for you."

Many Indians stopped using *ghee* and coconut oil for cooking because they heard that too much dietary fats led to heart disease. But two large meta-analyses since 2009 concluded there was not enough evidence to support this hypothesis. Thus, it is *not* likely that eating a *moderate* amount (roughly 2 tablespoons) of *ghee* or coconut oil each day will increase your risk of heart disease. Furthermore, *ghee* and coconut oil are ideal for cooking because they tend not to break down as easily as other common oils.

2. "There is not enough protein in a typical Indian diet."

Legumes (i.e., pulses) like *dal* and *channa* (chickpeas) are plentiful in Indian diets. When combined with whole grain foods like *chappatis*, you get all your essential amino acids. Snacking on nuts most days will ensure you get enough protein. If you like meat, preparing meat with Indian foods will also ensure you get enough protein, plus the other benefits of a healthy Indian diet.

115

3. "I get so many vegetables in my *subzi* every night, so I must be eating healthy."

Many Indian dishes are made by deep-frying vegetables or cooking them in excess heat. This destroys most of the vitamins and other phytonutrients, so your body won't get the benefits of these plant foods. To prevent this from happening, sauté or flash boil them. Or, if you must have your deep-fried dishes, eat raw plants by having fresh salads with your meals.

NOTE TO INDIAN AND SOUTH ASIAN READERS

What many of us Indians living in America eat is quite different than what generations before us ate. Nutrition-poor refined grains and fried vegetables have made their way into many of our daily diets. White rice as well as sugary or salty snacks are also common. Generally, there are less fresh plants in our diets, foods that control inflammation and the glucose/insulin feedback system.

In the past, people ate foods closer to how they were found in nature. The rice was brown or wild, other grains like millet and wheat were coarsely ground by stone milling, and thus much of the nutrition-rich bran and germ were included. *Dahi* was made from raw, unpasteurized milk fresh from the cow. Fruits and nuts were snacks, not chips and cookies. Dishes full of spices more often made their way into people's stomachs.

Along with changes to diet, levels of physical activity have also decreased. In the past, people walked every day to get around, whether to work, school, market, or home. People rarely walk this much anymore. These sweeping changes, especially to what Indian people eat, have had a large impact on health.

You may be aware anecdotally that more people in your community suffer from heart disease, diabetes, and cancers. Likely, you have observed that many middle-aged Indian men and women seem to have developed excessive belly fat. You may have recently learned of a new person, personally or through your network of friends and family, that has died from a heart attack, developed cancer, or suffered the complications of diabetes.

INDIANS SUFFER MORE CHRONIC DISEASES

Statistics on Indian people and their health certainly tell this story. According to Dr. Sunita Dodani at the Medical College of Georgia, "South Asians and [South Asian immigrants] have a much higher prevalence of diabetes, insulin resistance, central obesity, dyslipidemias ([low good cholesterol, high lipoprotein(a) and bad cholesterol, and high triglyceride]), [and] increased thrombotic tendency [or stickiness of the blood]," and metabolic syndrome (which is linked to coronary heart disease and diabetes).[181]

A PricewaterhouseCoopers report says that one of every 2 deaths in India today is due to chronic diseases, mostly heart disease, diabetes, and cancers.[182] By the year 2020, two of every 3 deaths in India will be caused by a chronic disease. Researchers writing in the *Lancet* predicted that 60% of the world's cardiovascular burden would be in India between 2008 and 2010.[183]

Dr. Milan Gupta and his collaborators wrote that people from the Indian Subcontinent have a 3 to 5-fold increase in the risk of heart attacks and cardiovascular deaths, and that they develop atherosclerotic disease at a greater rate by the age of 40 than any other people.[184] Explanations for poor health among South Asians include how our blood contains smaller LDL particles and higher levels of lipoprotein(a), which is similar to LDL-cholesterol, compared with other peoples. The combination of our genes and a Modern diet is behind why Indians have a higher rate of heart disease.[185]

The vulnerability of Indians due to the combination of genetics and a modern environment is also illustrated by the higher rates of diabetes. One study showed that South Asians who moved to America were more likely to develop insulin resistance, heart disease, and diabetes compared with American whites, blacks, and Hispanics.[186] Another showed that one South Asian person in every 6 in New York City has diabetes.[187] South Asian immigrants are more likely to develop diabetes compared with Caucasians in Britain.[188]

Diabetes is so prevalent that some experts say the BMI cutoff for what defines obesity (which is intimately linked to type 2 diabetes) should be *lowered* for South Asians from 30 kg/m² to 25 kg/m². Doing this would help doctors intervene on at-risk South Asians earlier.[189] Similar to heart disease, diabetes has been affecting more people in India too. Projections are that the number of diabetes cases in India will rise by 200%, to 57 million people, by 2025.[190] While people of Indian descent are likely to be genetically vulnerable to diabetes, a bigger factor is the broad changes to what people are eating.

Just as with heart disease and diabetes, metabolic syndrome is common among Indians. A 2009 review stated that 20% to 25% of South Asians have metabolic syndrome.[191] Some experts blamed the high prevalence on a diet high on easily digestible carbohydrates and fats and low on nutrition (i.e., the Modern diet), as well as people being more sedentary.[192]

There is at least one bright spot in terms of health for people of Indian descent: Cancers. For many common forms like lung cancer, Indians have relatively lower rates than people in Western counties. A large-scale survey demonstrated that people in India have lower rates of most cancers compared with Indians in Singapore, Britain, and America.[193] The exceptions to this rule are head and neck cancers, which are prevalent in India because more people have processed tobacco in *paan* (betel leaf) and cigarettes. Immigrant South Asians have lower rates compared with their white American counterparts.

Perhaps the fact that there are more plants – thus more anti-inflammatory phytonutrients – in the typical (even modern) Indian diet protects many Indian people against cancers. Better yet, the daily consumption of spices, including turmeric, black pepper, and ginger, deserves praise. Still, cancer rates among all people of Indian descent are rising.[194] What's to blame? The genes haven't changed after all, but the diet has.

THE MODERN INDIAN DIET IS TO BLAME

Simply, the modern Indian diet has too much sugar, white rice, white potatoes, and other forms of easily digestible carbohydrates. Eating this regularly will lead to insulin resistance in many people, and this will in turn lead to diabetes and heart disease. Not having many fresh plant and fermented foods keeps the general inflammation abnormally elevated, increasing the risk of developing chronic diseases. Experts are beginning to recognize this.

For example, doctors at India's Center for Diabetes, Obesity, and Cholesterol wrote in the *Journal of the American College of Nutrition* that Indians have gone from eating "a healthy traditional high-fiber, low-fat, low-calorie diet" to eating "calorie-dense foods containing refined carbohydrates, fats, red meats, and low fiber."[195] Others wrote that the high heart disease and insulin resistance rates in South Asians is due to there being too few monounsaturated fats – omega-3 fatty acids – and fiber in the diet, and too many saturated fats, carbs, and trans fats.[196]

Researchers who followed 1,800 Chennai (Madras) residents concluded that a diet high in foods with high Glycemic Loads (e.g., easily digestible carbohydrates) and low in fiber led to an increased risk of diabetes.[197] Early as 1994, the *New York Times* quoted researchers as saying that the consumption of easily digestible carbohydrates like sugar and bad fats (i.e., trans fats) explained why so many South Asians were developing heart disease, diabetes, and insulin resistance at higher rates than Americans and Europeans.[198]

Just as the carbohydrate hypothesis is gaining wider acceptance in the scientific community, and as the easily digestible carbohydrate is being blamed for the rising rates of obesity, coronary heart disease, insulin resistance, diabetes, and some cancers in the U.S., this bad form of carbohydrates is being blamed for the rising rates of chronic disease among Indians both in India and in the West.

IT IS EASY TO MAKE THE INDIAN DIET HEALTHIER

Genes certainly play some role, but unfortunately we can't control them. We can, however, control what we eat to a large extent. Based on historical evidence and the latest science, I have covered as well as possible what makes a healthy Indian diet. I hope you clearly understand that modern diets are the greatest *controllable* reason why so many people develop diabetes, heart disease and some cancers. From this, I hope you are inspired to focus on making what you eat healthier.

The dietary changes to improve your long-term health and avoid heart attacks, strokes, diabetes, and some cancers are simple. Eat less refined grains (e.g., *maida*) when cooking Indian food. Use more *atta* and other whole grain or chickpea flours instead. Eat more fresh vegetables. Eat fruits instead of sugary sweets, and heart-healthy nuts and peanuts instead of savory fried snacks. Use *ghee*, coconut oil, or canola oil for cooking. Add extra-virgin olive oil as a dressing (but never use it to cook vegetables).

Have *dahi* regularly, or some pickle or chutney made from fermentation. In all cases, cut down on sugar and salt. Eat more natural foods and foods that are close to how they are found in nature, and less of foods that are processed, overly milled, manufactured, and pre-packaged. There are a few other minor points covered in this book, but that is pretty much all there is to it.

PART III

HEALTHY

INDIAN RECIPES

VEGETARIAN DISHES

VEGETABLE JALFREZI – VEGETABLE STIR FRY

Vegetable *Jalfrezi* originated in India during the British Raj. Once a creative way to use up leftovers, the Vegetable *Jalfrezi* recipe has since evolved into a flavorful and texture-rich dish that is popular in Indian restaurants. Try this recipe with a mixture of vegetables or highlight just one or two. Either way, Vegetable *Jalfrezi* will add a colorful splash to your plate.

Prep Time: 15 minutes
Cook Time: 20 minutes
Serves: 4-5

Ingredients:

Cauliflower – 3 cups, cut into bite-sized florets
Carrots – ½ cup, chopped
Bell pepper – ½, cut into bite-sized pieces
Frozen green peas – ½ cup, thawed
Medium pot of water
Salt – 1 tsp
Turmeric powder – ¼ tsp
Canola Oil – 1 tbsp
Onion – ½ medium, chopped
Ginger – 1 tsp, minced
Garlic – 2 tsp, minced
Tomato Sauce – ½ cup (4 oz)
Salt – to taste
Whole coriander seeds – 2 tbsp, dry roasted and powdered
Garam masala – 1 tsp
Red chili powder – optional and to taste

Tomato – 1 small, deseeded and chopped

Lemon/lime juice – to taste

Method:

1. Bring pot of water to a boil and add salt and turmeric powder.

2. Add cauliflower and carrots. Boil for 3 minutes.

3. Strain vegetables and drop them in a bowl of ice water to stop further cooking.

4. Drain vegetables and keep aside for 1-2 minutes.

5. Heat oil in a medium non-stick skillet on medium heat.

6. Cook onions for 2-3 minutes until light golden.

7. Add ginger and garlic and sauté for 1 minute.

8. Add tomato sauce and cook until oil separates from the mixture.

9. Add bell pepper and green peas. Cook for 2-3 minutes.

10. Add cauliflower, carrots, salt, coriander powder, *garam masala* and red chili powder.

11. Mix and cook just until veggies are tender but not mushy.

12. Sprinkle a little water over the veggies occasionally to provide moisture and avoid burning.

13. Add tomato, mix and cook 1-2 minutes.

14. Sprinkle lemon/lime juice, mix and serve with paratha.

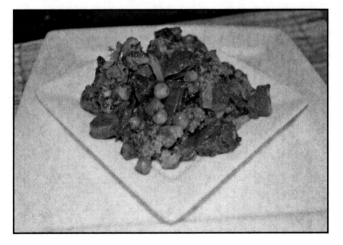

SHAHI PANEER – CHEESE CHUNKS IN CASHEW SAUCE

Shahi Paneer is a dish fit for a king. Paneer, homemade cheese, is cooked in a rich and creamy sauce made from cashews. Try this delectable and flavorful Indian dish that is also a restaurant favorite.

Prep Time: 15 minutes
Cook Time: 40 minutes
Serves: 6-8

Ingredients:

Paneer – 14oz block (homemade or store bought), cubed
Oil – 3 tbsp
Onions – 2 small, finely copped
Tomato sauce – 1, 8oz can
Garlic – 3 cloves, finely chopped
Ginger – 1 tbsp, minced
Green chilies – to taste, finely chopped
Cumin powder – 2 tsp
Coriander powder – 2 tsp
Garam masala – 2 tsp
Cashew pieces – ¾ cup
Milk – 1 cup
Water – 1 ½ cup
Sugar – 1 tbsp
Salt – to taste
Cilantro – 5 sprigs, finely chopped for garnishing

Method:

1. Soak cashews in milk for 15 minutes.
2. Meanwhile, heat 2 tbsp oil in a pan on medium to high heat.
3. Add onions and cook until translucent.
4. Add ginger, garlic, green chilies and cook until onions are golden brown.

5. Add tomato sauce and stir well. Cook until oil separates from the mixture.

6. Blend soaked cashews and milk until smooth and keep aside.

7. To the cooked onion/tomato sauce mixture, add cumin powder, coriander powder and *garam masala*. Mix well.

8. Add blended cashews and milk and mix until there are no lumps in the gravy.

9. Add water, salt and sugar and bring to a boil.

10. In a separate pan, sauté *paneer* in 1 tbsp of oil on medium to high heat until light golden brown. Remove onto a paper towel lined plate.

11. Once gravy comes to the boil, add *paneer* and mix.

12. Garnish with fresh cilantro or with additional broken cashew pieces.

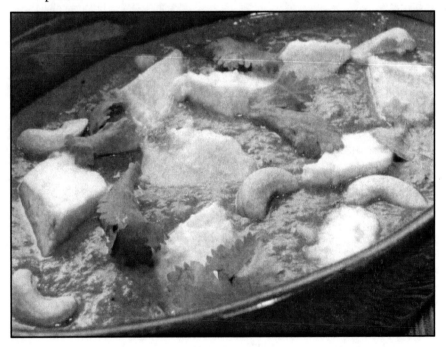

ASPARAGUS SUBZI – ASPARAGUS SIDE DISH

Asparagus is not usually associated with Indian cooking. The long bright-green spears have tender tips while the tough ends are discarded. Asparagus is a nutrient-rich food that is high in folic acid and a good source of potassium, fiber, vitamin B6, vitamins A and C and thiamin. Many people tend to overlook this delicious vegetable due to lack of know-how in the preparation stage. Now, you can try fresh and tender Asparagus – the Indian way!

Prep time: 10 minutes
Cook Time: 10 minutes
Serves: 4

Ingredients:

Asparagus – 1 lb, chopped into bite-sized pieces
Canola oil – 1 tbsp
Cumin seeds – ½ tsp
Fennel seeds (powdered) – ½ tsp
Ginger – 1 tsp, grated or crushed
Garlic – 5 large cloves, roughly chopped
Tomatoes – 2 medium, chopped
Salt – to taste
Red chili powder – to taste

Method:

1. Wash asparagus and snap the white/hard ends and discard.
2. Chop into bite-sized pieces.
3. In a skillet, heat oil on medium heat.
4. Add cumin seeds and allow them to splutter.
5. Add powdered fennel seeds, ginger and garlic and cook for a minute.
6. Add tomatoes and cook until soft.
7. Add asparagus, salt and red chili powder. Mix well.

8.   Cook uncovered for 5-6 minutes until moisture has evaporated.

9.   Serve hot with paratha.

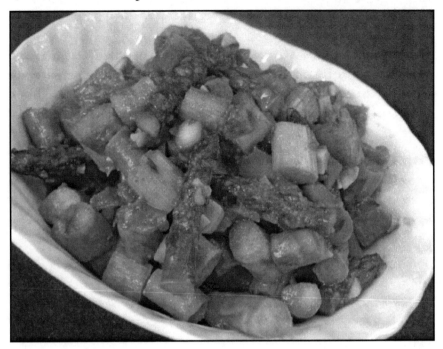

KUMRO CHOKKA – BUTTERNUT SQUASH WITH BLACK CHICKPEAS

The varying textures and contrasting colors of this Bengali recipe provide a visual feast for the eyes. The sweetness from the butternut squash is perfectly balanced with the earthy goodness of the black chickpeas. This delicious and fiber-rich dish is sure to be a family favorite.

Prep Time: 10 minutes plus minimum 8 hours soaking time
Cook Time: 1 hour
Serves: 4-6

Ingredients:

Butternut squash (or pumpkin) – 1 ½ lbs (peeled, seeds and fiber removed and cubed into bite-sized pieces)
Black Chickpeas (*Kala Chana*, dry) – 1 cup
Water – 3 cups
Salt – to taste
Canola oil – 2 tbsp
Panch phoron – 1 tsp (see below for recipe)
Red chili powder – to taste
Cumin powder – 1 tsp
Ginger – 1 tbsp, minced
Sugar or jaggery or brown sugar – 1 tsp, optional and to taste

Method:

1. Wash chickpeas and soak in water overnight (minimum 8 hrs).
2. Rinse chickpeas and transfer them to a pressure cooker.
3. Add 3 cups water and salt (½ tbsp or to taste).
4. Pressure cook on high heat for 1 whistle (or 1-2 minutes after full pressure is attained), reduce heat to low and continue cooking for 30 minutes.
5. Remove from heat and do not open pressure cooker until all internal pressure is released.

6. Drain liquid from chickpeas and set them aside.
7. Heat oil in a medium pan on medium heat.
8. Add panch phoron and allow the seeds to pop and sizzle.
9. Add squash, mix well, cover and cook until three quarters done (approximately 12 minutes). Stir periodically for even cooking. Squash should be translucent and soft but not mushy.
10. Add salt, red chili powder, cumin powder, ginger and sugar. Mix well and cook for 2-3 minutes.
11. Add drained chickpeas, mix well, and adjust spices to taste. Cook until squash is fully tender.

Panch Puran Recipe: (mix equal portions of each)

Fenugreek seeds, cumin seeds, mustard seeds, nigella seeds (kalonji) and fennel seeds.

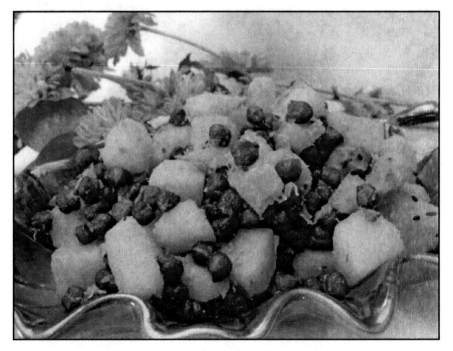

BAINGAN KI SUBZI – ROASTED EGGPLANT SIDE DISH

"Simple" is the perfect way to describe this no-frills eggplant dish made by roasting eggplant and adding a few ingredients that are always on hand. It's a perfect way to "hide" vegetables for picky eaters.

Prep Time: 1 hour
Cook Time: 10 minutes
Serves: 3-4

Ingredients:

Eggplant – 1 lb
Canola oil – 1 tbsp
Asafoetida – ⅛ tsp (optional)
Onion – ½ large
Garlic – 1 tbsp, minced
Green chilies – to taste, finely chopped
Turmeric powder – 1/4 tsp
Salt – to taste
Lime/lemon juice – to taste
Cilantro – 10 sprigs, finely chopped

Method:

1. Pre-heat oven to 400 degrees Fahrenheit (approximately 200 degrees Celsius).
2. Line a baking pan with foil.
3. Coat entire eggplant with a little oil and bake it for 1 hour.
4. Remove pan from oven and allow eggplant to cool down to touch.
5. Cut off stem and peel the skin off of eggplant. Discard both.
6. Transfer flesh to another bowl and roughly chop it.
7. Heat oil in a medium pan on medium heat.
8. Add asafoetida (optional), onions, garlic, green chilies and turmeric powder.

9. Add salt, mix well and allow onions to cook until translucent (approximately 3-5 minutes).
10. Add eggplant and allow it to heat all the way through.
11. Add lemon/lime juice and cilantro. Mix well.
12. Serve hot with *paratha*.

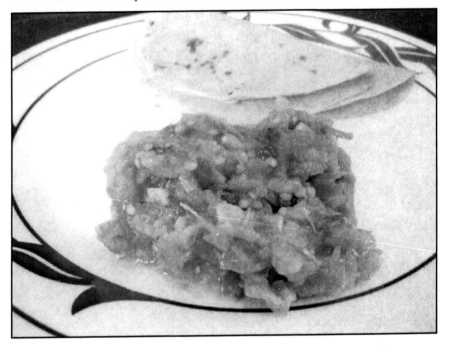

CHANA MASALA (OR CHOLE) – GARBANZO BEANS CURRY

Garbanzo beans (*kabuli chana*) belong to the class of food called legumes and are an excellent source of protein and both soluble and insoluble fiber. This recipe for *Chana Masala* showcases this nutty, buttery bean in a tangy and flavorful tomato based sauce.

Prep Time: 5 minutes + overnight soaking
Cook Time: 60 minutes
Serves: 6-8

Ingredients:

Garbanzo beans (dry) – 2 cups
Water – 6 cups (more as needed)
Tea bags – 2
Black cardamom – 1
Bay leaf – 1
Cinnamon stick – 1-inch piece
Salt – to taste
Canola oil – 1 ½ tbsp
Asafoetida – ⅛ tsp
Crushed tomatoes – 2 cups or 14 ½ oz can
Chana/chole masala – 1 tbsp
Dried pomegranate seeds (*Anardana*) – ½ tsp, powdered
Red chili powder – ½ tsp
Chaat masala – ½ tsp
Dry mango powder (*Amchur*) – ½ tsp
Onions & green chilies – for garnishing

Method:

1. Soak garbanzo beans in 6 cups of water overnight or for at least 8 hours.
2. Transfer them along with the water into a pressure cooker.
3. Add cinnamon stick, bay leaf, black cardamom, teabags and salt.

134

4.   Mix and pressure-cook on medium/high heat for 3 whistles (or for 3 minutes after cooker attains full pressure).

5.   Reduce heat to low and continue cooking for an additional 20 minutes.

6.   Remove from heat and do not open pressure cooker until all internal pressure is released.

7.   Remove the garbanzo beans from the liquid and keep aside. Do not discard the liquid.

8.   In a pan, heat oil on medium heat.

9.   Add asafoetida and crushed tomatoes.

10. Cook until the tomatoes clump together and separate from the oil.

11. Add chana masala, chaat masala, red chili powder, dry mango powder & anardana powder. Mix well.

12. Add cooked garbanzo beans and mix again.

13. Add reserved liquid, cover and cook until desired consistency is attained.

14. Garnish with onions and green chilies and serve hot with Indian flatbread or brown rice.

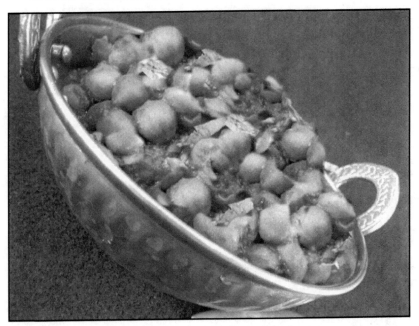

Lauki Koftas – Bottle Gourd & Chickpea Flour Dumplings

Bottle gourd (also known as *lauki* or *dudhi*) is a vegetable renowned for its simplistic and mild flavor. Due to its high water content, bottle gourd offers a nutrient-filled but low-caloric option for those watching their weight. This recipe dresses up the low-key flavors of bottle gourd and provides a flavorful curry that's sure to please.

Prep time: 30 minutes
Cook time: 30 minutes
Serves: 6

Ingredients:

For the Koftas:

Bottle gourd – 4 cups (peeled & shredded)
Chickpea flour (*Besan*) – 3/4 cup
Onion – ¼ medium, finely chopped
Roasted peanuts – ¼ cup, roughly powdered
Cilantro – 10 sprigs, finely chopped
Coriander powder – 1 tsp
Cumin powder – ½ tsp
Dry Mango powder (*Amchur*) – ½ tsp
Garam masala – ½ tsp
Red Chili powder – to taste
Salt – to taste

For the Gravy:

Canola oil – 2 tbsp
Onions – 2 medium, minced
Salt – to taste
Garlic – 4 cloves, minced
Ginger – 1 tsp, minced
Green chilies – to taste, finely chopped

136

Tomatoes – 3 large, pureed
Coriander powder – 1 tsp
Cumin powder – ½ tsp
Garam masala – ¼ tsp
Yogurt (or *Dahi*) – ½ cup
Water – 3 ½ cups
Cilantro – for garnishing

Method:

1.   For the gravy, heat oil in a medium pan on medium heat.
2.   Add onions and sprinkle a little salt to speed up cooking process.
3.   Once moisture has evaporated from onions, add ginger, garlic and green chilies.
4.   Allow onions to turn golden brown before adding tomatoes.
5.   Cook until mixture clumps together and oil separates from the mixture.
6.   Add turmeric powder, cumin powder, coriander powder and *garam masala.*
7.   Mix well and add yogurt.
8.   Mix and add water to achieve desired consistency. Add Salt to taste.
9.   Cover and allow gravy to come to a boil.
10. For the koftas, squeeze out excess liquid from shredded bottle gourd and add liquid to gravy.
11. Place bottle gourd in a mixing bowl and add chickpea flour as needed (enough to form balls (koftas)).
12. Add peanuts, onions, cilantro, red chili powder, dry mango powder, cumin & coriander powders, *garam masala* and salt. Mix well to incorporate all ingredients.
13. Form balls (koftas) and drop them into boiling gravy. Pour gravy over the koftas if they are not fully submerged.
14. Increase heat to maintain the boil as koftas are added.
15. Cover and cook for 5 minutes, turning koftas over once in between if they are not fully submerged in the gravy.
16. Garnish with cilantro and serve hot with *paratha* (Indian flat bread).

SEM PHALI – LIMA BEAN CURRY

Though lima beans (also known as butter beans) are often overlooked, it's hard to miss how rich they are in basic nutrition. Lima beans provide virtually fat-free high-quality protein and a great source of cholesterol-lowering fiber. Try this flavorful dish and thank yourself for giving this unique bean a second taste.

Prep Time: 10 minutes
Cook Time: 30 minutes
Serves: 4

Ingredients:

Frozen lima beans – 16oz packet (rinsed)
Canola oil – 1 tbsp + 1 tsp
Cumin seeds – ½ tsp
Mustard seeds – ½ tsp
Asafoetida – ⅛ tsp
Turmeric powder – ¼ tsp
Onion – 1 small, finely chopped
Green chili – 1, finely chopped (optional)
Ginger – 1 tsp, finely grated
Garlic – 3 cloves, finely chopped
Tomato sauce – 8oz can
Red chili powder – ¼ tsp (to taste)
Coriander powder – 1 tsp
Garam masala – 1 tsp
Cumin powder – ½ tsp
Salt – 1 tsp (to taste)
Water – 1 cup
Cilantro leaves – 5 sprigs, chopped for garnishing
Lime juice – optional for garnishing

Method:

138

1. Heat oil in a pressure cooker on medium heat.
2. Once oil is hot, add cumin seeds and mustard seeds and allow them to splutter.
3. Add asafoetida and turmeric powder, then onions, green chili, ginger and garlic.
4. Cook until onions are light brown.
5. Stir in tomato sauce and cook until oil starts to separate from the mixture.
6. Add red chili powder, coriander powder, *garam masala*, cumin powder, and salt. Mix well and cook for 1-2 minutes.
7. Mix in lima beans and water.
8. Pressure cook for 1 whistle (or for 1-2 minutes after full pressure is attained). Remove from heat and do not open pressure cooker until all internal pressure is released.
9. Adjust water, salt or other spices.
10. Garnish with cilantro and lime juice and serve with brown rice or paratha.

Note: This recipe can be prepared without a pressure cooker. Microwave lima beans with ½ cup water, salt and turmeric powder. Follow steps 1-6 and mix in cooked lima beans and additional water. Bring to a boil and cook for 5-7 minutes.

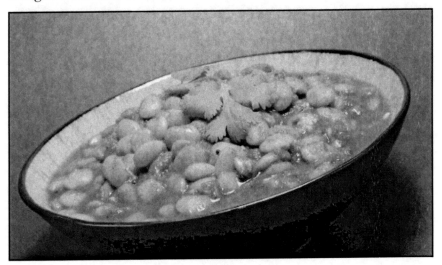

DAL-BASED (LENTIL) SOUPS

TADKA DAL FRY

Tadka Dal Fry is a wonderful combination of 3 different lentils (*dals*). The amazing flavors will have everyone guessing which *dal* they are enjoying. Blend it well for a smooth texture or leave it as is for a rustic treat.

Prep Time: 10 minutes + 20 minutes for soaking
Cook time: 30 minutes
Serves: 4

Ingredients:

Split pigeon peas (*Toor Dal*) – ⅓ cup
Split mung without skin (*Mung Dal*) – ⅓ cup
Split chickpeas (*Chana Dal*) – ⅓ cup
Water – 3 cups
Canola oil – 1 tbsp
Onion – 1 medium, finely chopped
Turmeric powder – ¼ tsp
Cumin powder – ½ tsp
Coriander powder – 1 tsp
Garam masala – ½ tsp
Red chili powder – to taste
Salt – to taste

For Tadka (Seasoning):

Clarified butter (ghee) – 2 tsp
Mustard seeds – ½ tsp
Cumin seeds – ½ tsp
Asafoetida – ⅛ tsp
Curry leaves – few

140

Garlic – 2 cloves, finely chopped

Ginger – 1 tsp, grated

Green chili – to taste, slit

Lime juice – to taste, for garnishing

Cilantro – finely chopped, for garnishing

Method:

1. Combine all *dals*, wash them well and soak for 20-30 minutes.
2. Drain off water and add soaked *dals* to a pressure cooker.
3. Add water and salt.
4. Pressure cook on medium heat for 3 whistles or 3 minutes after full pressure is attained. Remove from heat and do not open pressure cooker until all internal pressure is released.
5. Meanwhile, heat oil in a medium pan on medium heat.
6. Add turmeric powder and asafoetida.
7. Add onions and a little salt and cook until onions are translucent.
8. Add cumin powder, red chili powder, coriander powder and *garam masala*. Cook for 10-15 seconds.
9. Stir in cooked *dal* and adjust salt and water to desired consistency.
10. Bring to a boil and cook for 4-5 minutes.
11. Pour *dal* in a serving dish and set aside.
12. For the *tadka* (seasoning), heat clarified butter in a small skillet on medium heat.
13. Add mustard seeds and allow them to pop.
14. Add cumin seeds, curry leaves, green chilies, garlic, ginger and cook for 1 minute.
15. Pour seasoning over *dal* and garnish with cilantro leaves and lime juice.

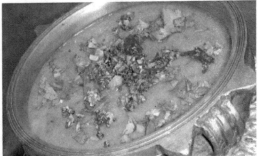

WHOLE GREEN MUNG DAL – MUNG BEAN SOUP

Mung (or *Moong*) beans, with their green outer husk intact, are a rich source of fiber and calcium and more easily digested than other beans. This wholesome, hearty *Mung Dal* recipe is packed with protein, and eating it with brown rice or just by itself as a soup is wonderfully comforting!

Prep Time: 4 hours for soaking Mung Beans
Cook Time: 30 minutes
Serves: 4

Ingredients:

Whole mung beans (dry) – 1 cup
Water – 3 cups
Salt – to taste
Canola oil – 1 tbsp
Cumin seeds – ½ tsp
Asafoetida – ⅛ tsp
Turmeric powder – ¼ tsp
Garlic cloves – 4 large, roughly crushed
Ginger – ½ tbsp, grated
Curry leaves – few leaves
Green chilies – to taste, slit
Tomato – 1 medium, chopped
Cilantro – 5 sprigs, chopped
Lemon/lime juice – to taste

Method:

1. Wash and soak whole green mung beans in ample water for about 4 hours.
2. Drain water and rinse beans.
3. Add soaked mung beans, 3 cups water and salt to a pressure cooker.

4. Pressure cook for 1 whistle or 1-2 minute after full pressure is attained. Remove from heat and do not open pressure cooker until all internal pressure is released.
5. Heat oil in a medium pot on medium heat.
6. Add Cumin seeds and allow them to sizzle.
7. Add asafoetida, turmeric powder, curry leaves, ginger, garlic and green chilies. Cook for 30 seconds.
8. Add tomatoes and cook for 1 minute, just until soft.
9. Add cooked mung, bring to a boil, then reduce heat to a simmer for a few minutes.
10. Adjust salt, add lime juice and garnish with cilantro (coriander leaves).

DAL MAKHANI – BLACK GRAM LEGUME SOUP

Dal Makhani, made with whole *Urad Dal* (black gram), is an Indian restaurant staple dish. It is known by many different names, including *Kaali* (Black) *Dal* and *Maa ki Dal*. *Dal Makhani* gained popularity in India as typical *dhaaba* (roadside stand) fare but has made its way into homes with its fantastic flavor and rustic charm.

Soaking Time: Overnight or minimum 8 hours
Prep Time: 10 minutes
Cook Time: 45 minutes
Serves: 4-6

Ingredients:

Whole black gram (whole *urad* with skin, dry) – 1 cup
Kidney beans (dry) – ¼ cup
Water – 3 cups
Onion – ½ medium, chopped
Garlic – 1 tsp, minced
Ginger – 1 tsp, minced
Green chili – to taste, chopped or slit
Salt – to taste
Coriander powder – 1 tsp
Cumin powder – ½ tsp
Turmeric powder – ¼ tsp
Garam masala – 1 tsp
Red chili powder – to taste
Yogurt – 2 tbsp (well beaten)
Heavy whipping cream – 3 tbsp
Canola oil – 1 tbsp
Cumin seeds – ½ tsp
Tomato – 1 medium, chopped
Additional cream or butter for garnishing

Method:

1. Wash whole black gram and kidney beans well and soak overnight in the 3 cups of water.
2. Add soaked beans into a pressure cooker along with the water.
3. Add *garam masala*, coriander powder, cumin powder, turmeric powder, red chili powder, onions, green chili, salt, ginger and garlic.
4. Mix well and pressure cook for 3 whistles (or 3-4 minutes after full pressure is attained).
5. Lower flame and simmer for 20 minutes.
6. Remove from heat and do not open until all internal pressure is released.
7. Carefully open pressure cooker and stir. Dal should be soft and cooked well.
8. Turn on stove to low heat and allow *dal* to come to a boil.
9. Add yogurt and cream and keep cooking on low flame.
10. For the seasoning, heat oil in a small skillet on medium heat.
11. Add cumin seeds and allow them to sizzle.
12. Add tomatoes and cook until soft (do not overcook).
13. Add seasoning to *dal* and gently mix.
14. Garnish with a additional cream or a knob of butter.

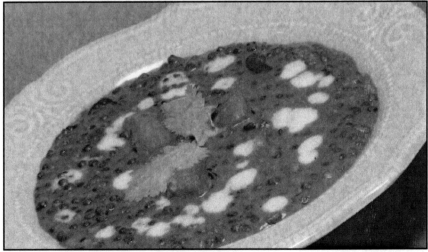

SAMBAR – SOUTH INDIAN LEGUME SOUP

Sambar is a staple dish in most South Indian meals. Every family has its own personal touch when making this versatile *dal*. *Sambar* is a perfect complement to *Dosa* or *Idli*.

Prep time: 30 minutes
Cook time: 30 minutes
Serves: 4-6

Ingredients:

Split pigeon peas (*Toor Dal*) – 1 cup
Water – 3+1 cup
Tindora – 5 to 6, julienned
Carrot – 1, cut to bite-sized pieces
Green beans – ¼ cup, cut into 1-inch pieces
Winter melon/ash gourd – ½ cup, cubed
Salt – to taste
Tamarind pulp – 1 to 1 ½ tbsp or to taste (tamarind concentrate may be used in lesser quantity)
Asafoetida – ¼ tsp (divided)
Turmeric powder – ¼ tsp
Red chili powder – to taste (divided)
Sambar powder – 4 tsp (divided)
Tomato – ½ medium, cubed
Canola oil – 1 ½ tbsp
Mustard seeds – 1 tsp
Curry leaves – 1 sprig
Coriander powder – 1 tbsp
Cilantro/coriander leaves – for garnishing

Method:

1.   Wash and soak the *Toor Dal* for 30 minutes.
2.   Drain water and add *Toor Dal* to a pressure cooker.

3. Add carrots, green beans, tindora, winter melon, water (3 cups) and salt.

4. Cook *dal* on medium heat until pressure cooker whistles once (or 1-2 minutes after full pressure is attained).

5. Remove from heat and do not open pressure cooker until all internal pressure is released.

6. Meanwhile, soak dry tamarind in ½ cup hot water and allow it to soften.

7. Open pressure cooker and return it to the stove on medium heat.

8. Add turmeric powder, tomatoes, ⅛ tsp asafoetida, ½ chili powder and ½ *sambar* powder.

9. Mix well and allow *sambar* to keep boiling.

10. Mash tamarind to extract pulp from fiber and seeds. Use a sieve and strain pulp into boiling *sambar*.

11. Add additional water (1 cup or as needed) for desired *sambar* consistency. Boil for 5 minutes.

12. For the seasoning, Heat oil in a small skillet on medium heat.

13. Add mustard seeds and ⅛ tsp asafoetida. allow mustard seeds to pop.

14. Add curry leaves and remove skillet from stove.

15. Add remaining red chili powder and *sambar* powder and coriander powder. Mix quickly and add ¼ cup water to prevent spices from burning.

16. Add seasoning to *sambar*, mix and allow it to boil for another 2-3 minutes.

17. Garnish with cilantro (coriander leaves).

DAAR – GUJARATI LENTIL SOUP

Gujarati *Daar* (dal) has a perfect balance of flavors – A hint of sweetness from the jaggery, tartness from the *kokum* and the heat from the spices and green chilies! Combined with brown rice, Gujarati *Daar* is the ultimate end to a traditional Gujarati *thali* (meal).

Prep Time: 25 minutes (including soaking time)
Cook Time: 30 minutes (plus time for boiling)
Serves: 6-8

Ingredients:

Split pigeon peas (*Toor Dal*) – 1½ cups (washed, soaked for 20 minutes)
Water – 4 ½ cups for pressure cooking
Raw peanuts – ½ cup
Fenugreek seeds – ⅛ tsp
Salt – to taste
Turmeric powder – ¼ tsp
Water – 4 cups to thin *dal*
Red chili powder – ½ tsp or to taste
Coriander powder – 2 tsp
Cumin powder – 1 tsp
Garam masala – 1 tsp
Kokum – 3 to 4
Green chilies – 2 or to taste, finely chopped
Tomato – 1 medium, diced
Jaggery – 3 tbsp or to taste
Dry mango powder (*Amchur*) – 1 tsp
Ginger – 2 tsp, grated
Lemon/lime juice – 1 tbsp or to taste
Cilantro – 5 sprigs, chopped for garnishing

For the seasoning:

Canola oil – 2 tsp

Clarified butter (ghee) – 2 tsp
Mustard seeds – ½ tsp
Cumin seeds – ½ tsp
Fenugreek seeds – ⅛ tsp
Asafoetida – ⅛ tsp
Whole dried red chili – 1
Whole cloves – 4
Cinnamon stick – 1-inch piece
Curry leaves – 1 sprig

Method:

1. Drain soaked *Toor Dal.*
2. Cook in pressure cooker with water, fenugreek seeds, salt, peanuts and turmeric powder.
3. Pressure cook for 4-5 whistles (or 4-5 minutes after full pressure is attained).
4. Remove from heat and do not open pressure cooker until all internal pressure is released.
5. Open pressure cooker and return to stove on medium heat.
6. Add red chili powder, cumin powder, coriander powder, *garam masala, kokum,* green chilies, tomato, ginger and jaggery.
7. Mix well and add up to 4 cups of additional water, a little at a time, to get desired consistency.
8. Allow *dal* to boil for at least 10 minutes (boiling longer improves flavor).
9. For seasoning, heat oil and ghee in a small skillet.
10. Add mustard seeds and allow them to pop.
11. Add cumin seeds and allow them to sizzle.
12. Add fenugreek seeds, cloves, cinnamon stick, asafoetida, whole dried red chili and curry leaves. Mix and add seasoning to boiling *dal.*
13. Add lemon/lime juice and/or dry mango powder to desired tartness.
14. Adjust sweetness (jaggery), salt or any other spices to taste.
15. Garnish with cilantro and serve hot with plain rice, brown rice or paratha.

MEAT DISHES

DOI MAACH – BENGALI FISH CURRY

Doi Maach is a popular Bengali fish curry made with unmistakable and aromatic mustard oil. Rohu fish is used to get the authentic flavor but can be substituted with red snapper, halibut, cod, haddock or swordfish.

Prep Time: 5 minutes
Cook Time: 25 minutes
Serves: 2-3

Ingredients:

Rohu fish – ½ lb (substitutes: red snapper, halibut, cod, haddock, swordfish)
Turmeric powder – ¼ tsp + ¼ tsp
Salt – ¼ tsp + ¼ tsp or to taste
Onion – ½ medium, blended
Mustard oil – 3 tbsp
Cardamom – 4
Cloves – 4
Bay leaves – 2 to 3
Cinnamon – 1 inch piece
Green chilies – to taste, slit
Ginger – 1 tsp, minced
Red chili powder – to taste
Sugar – ¼ tsp
Yogurt – 2 tbsp
Water – 2 tbsp
Golden raisins – 1 tsp, optional
Water – 2 cups

Method:

1. Wash and clean fish.
2. Rub fish with ¼ tsp turmeric and ¼ tsp salt.
3. Allow fish to marinate for 5-10 minutes.
4. With a mortar and pestle, pound Cardamom and cloves and discard cardamom skin. Set aside.
5. Heat mustard oil in a medium pan on medium heat.
6. Lightly fry fish, one minute on each side. Do not over crowd pan. Remove fish onto a paper towel lined plate until ready to use.
7. In the same oil, add bay leaves, ground cloves and cardamom, onion paste, green chilies and ¼ tsp salt. Mix and cook for 2-3 minutes.
8. Add ginger, turmeric powder, red chili powder and sugar. Mix.
9. Dilute yogurt with 2 tbsp water and make a smooth paste. Turn off stove and slowly add yogurt to the pan, while stirring continuously.
10. Once yogurt is mixed in, turn stove on and add raisins.
11. Cook until oil separates from the mixture.
12. Gently add fish into the mixture and cook it on both sides for 1-2 minutes.
13. Add warm water (2 cups) and mix very gently to incorporated the mixture.
14. Reduce heat to low, cover and cook for 10 minutes.
15. Uncover, increase the heat to high and cook for another 5-7 minutes or until gravy is of desired consistency.
16. Serve with brown rice or *paratha*.

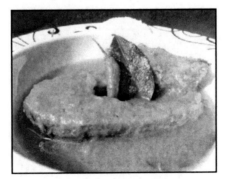

SAAGWALA MURGH – CHICKEN CURRY WITH SPINACH

This recipe is a great way to incorporate vegetables and protein into one dish. The flavor is mild yet satisfying. For those with taste buds that scream for hot and spicy dishes, just double the *garam masala*, red chili powder, and curry powder – an easy fix!

Prep Time: 10 minutes
Cook Time: 40 minutes
Serves: 6 to 8

Ingredients:

Chicken – 2 lbs, boneless, skinless thighs cut to bite-size pieces
Spinach – 16 oz, frozen chopped
Tomatoes – 6 medium, finely chopped
Canola oil – 4 tsp
Black cardamom – 1
Cinnamon – 1-inch piece
Green cardamom – 2
Bay leaves – 2
Cloves – 4
Onions – 1 large, finely chopped
Ginger – 2 tsp, minced
Garlic – 5 cloves, minced
Green chilies – to taste, finely chopped
Salt – to taste
Red chili powder – ½ tsp
Garam masala – 1 tsp
Cumin powder – 1 tsp
Coriander powder – 1 tsp
Curry powder – 1 tsp

Method:

1.   Heat oil in a medium pan on medium heat.

2. Add bay leaves, cloves, cinnamon and cardamom.

3. Add onions and a little salt and mix well. Cover and cook about 5 minutes (until onions turn translucent).

4. Add ginger, garlic, green chilies and tomatoes. Mix, cover and continue to cook until oil separates from the mixture. Stir in between.

5. Add chicken, cumin powder, coriander powder, salt, red chili powder, *garam masala* and curry powder. Mix well, cover and continue to cook for 5-7 minutes.

6. Add spinach, mix, cover and cook for approximately 10 minutes (until chicken is no longer pink from the inside).

7. Serve hot with paratha or brown rice.

GRAIN-BASED DISHES AND BREADS

OATS AND BROWN RICE DOSA – SAVORY SOUTH INDIAN CREPE

Contrary to popular belief, the ever-popular *dosa* can be made in a healthy way. Originally made with mostly white rice, this delicious recipe is made with power packed oats and the nutty texture of brown rice. Pair it with coconut chutney or *sambar* for a fantastic South Indian meal with a healthy twist.

Prep Time: 10 minutes (plus 8 hours soaking time)
Cooking Time: 2 minutes for each Dosa
Yields: Approximately 25 Dosas

Ingredients:

Instant (quick) oats – 3 cups
Long grain brown rice – 1 cup
Split black gram (*Urad Dal*) – 1 cup
Fenugreek seeds – 1 tsp
Salt – 2 tsp or to taste
Canola oil – for pan frying
Water – 1½ cups to grind brown rice and *dal* and 2½ cups to soak and grind oats

Method:

1. Wash brown rice and soak with fenugreek seeds in ample water overnight (minimum 8 hours).
2. An hour prior to grinding, soak Oats in 2 ½ cups water and wash and soak *urad dal* in ample water.
3. Drain water from brown rice and fenugreek seeds and using a blender, blend brown rice and fenugreek seeds with 1 cup fresh water. Transfer to a large bowl.

154

4. To the blender, add drained *urad dal* and ½ cup fresh water. Grind to smooth paste and transfer to large bowl.

5. Blend oats along with the soaking water until smooth. Transfer to large bowl.

6. Mix the batter (brown rice, *urad dal* and oats) very well, preferably with your hand, in one direction.

7. Cover bowl and allow the mixture to ferment in a warm place for 8-10 hours (no more).

8. After fermentation, transfer batter to refrigerator until ready to use.

9. To make dosas, add salt to batter and mix well.

10. Additional water may be needed to get batter to pouring consistency as oats tend to thicken over time.

11. Heat *tawa* or flat skillet on medium-high. Water must sizzle and evaporate immediately.

12. Once skillet is hot, drizzle a few drops of oil, coat surface and wipe off with a paper towel.

13. Pour a ladleful of batter in the center of the skillet and starting from the center, move ladle in a circular motion outwards to spread the batter.

14. Allow *dosa* to cook on bottom side.

15. When the batter dries, drizzle a few drops of oil and allow it to cook until color changes slightly.

16. Loosen edges of the *dosa* and flip it. Allow the other side to cook for 30 seconds.

17. Remove *dosa* from the skillet and serve immediately with *sambar* or chutney.

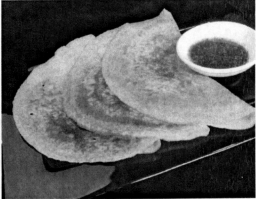

BASIC BROWN RICE

Brown rice has a wonderful nutty flavor and texture that is an enjoyable change from regular white rice, not to mention that it is also nutritionally superior compared to other varieties of rice. Try this delicious brown rice with any Indian curry – a break from the mundane.

Cook Time: 45-50 minutes
Serves: 4

Ingredients:

Brown Rice – 1 cup
Water – 2 cups
Salt – ½ tsp (optional)

Pressure Cooker Method:

1. Wash and drain brown rice.
2. Combine brown rice, salt and water in pressure cooker.
3. Pressure cook for 2 whistles on medium (or 2 minutes after full pressure is attained), reduce flame to low and cook for 30 minutes.
4. Remove from flame and do not open pressure cooker until all internal pressure is released.
5. Fluff brown rice gently with a fork.
6. Cover and allow it to rest 5 minutes. Serve hot.

Stove-top Method:

1. Wash and drain brown rice.
2. In a pan, combine brown rice, salt and water.
3. On medium flame, bring to a boil.
4. Reduce heat to a low, cover with tight lid and cook for 45 minutes.

5. Remove from heat and fluff gently with a fork.
6. Cover and allow it to rest 5 minutes. Serve hot.

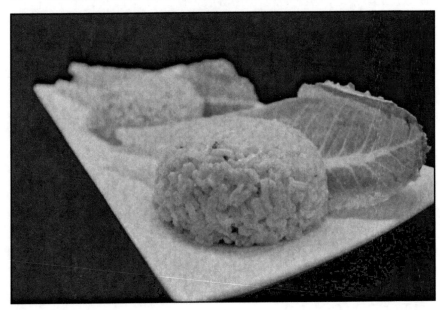

MASALA BROWN RICE – SPICED BROWN RICE

This recipe takes left-over basic brown rice to a flavor high point. It is delicious enough to make brown rice from scratch just to taste this fabulous makeover.

Prep Time: 5 minutes
Cook Time: 7 minutes
Serves: 2-3

Ingredients:

Cooked brown rice – 3 cups
Canola oil – 1 tbsp
Mustard seeds – ½ tsp
Asafoetida – ⅛ tsp
Turmeric powder – ¼ tsp
Raw peanuts – 3 tbsp
Curry leaves – sprig
Green chilies – to taste, finely chopped
Chana masala – 2 tsp or to taste
Salt – to taste
Cilantro – for garnish

Method:

1. Warm leftover brown rice in microwave to room temperature.
2. Add *chana masala* and salt to brown rice and mix well. Keep aside.
3. Heat oil in a medium pan on medium heat.
4. Add mustard seeds and allow them to pop.
5. Add asafoetida and turmeric powder.
6. Add peanuts and allow them to cook until golden in color. (Tip: use roasted peanuts to reduce cooking time.)
7. Add curry leaves, green chilies and brown rice.
8. Mix well and allow brown rice to heat all the way through.

9.   Garnish with fresh cilantro and serve hot.

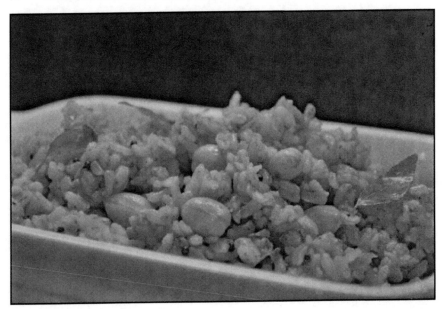

QUINOA PULAO – QUINOA PILAF

Quinoa is a grain-like crop often referred to as a complete protein. (Grains, on the other hand, do not contain complete proteins and thus must be combined with lentils or *dals*.) Quinoa has cooking properties similar to white rice and can easily be used as a healthy substitute, as seen in this recipe for Quinoa Pulao.

Prep Time: 10 minutes (plus 30 minutes for soaking)
Cook Time: 50 minutes
Serves: 4 to 6

Ingredients:

Quinoa – 2 cups
Canola oil – 2 tbsp
Bay leaf – 1
Cinnamon – 1-inch piece
Black cardamom -1
Green cardamom – 2
Black pepper – 4 or to taste, roughly crushed
Cloves – 4, roughly crushed
Turmeric powder – ¼ tsp
Onion – ½ medium, finely chopped
Ginger – 1 tbsp, minced
Garlic – 1 tbsp, minced
Green chilies – to taste, finely chopped
Corn – 1 cup
Green peas – 1 cup
Carrots – 1 cup, chopped
Garam masala – 1 tsp
Coriander powder – 1 tsp
Cumin powder – ½ tsp
Salt – to taste

Water – 3 cups
Lemon/lime juice – to taste
Cilantro – chopped for garnishing

Method:

1. Wash quinoa and soak in ample water for 30 minutes.
2. Drain water and set quinoa aside.
3. Heat oil in a medium pan on medium heat.
4. Add bay leaf, cinnamon stick, black cardamom and green cardamom. Cook for 30 seconds.
5. Add black pepper, cloves and cumin seeds. Allow them to sizzle.
6. Add turmeric powder and onions. Cook for 1 minute.
7. Add ginger, garlic and green chilies. Mix well and cook until onions are translucent.
8. Add quinoa and roast for 5 minutes.
9. Add corn, green peas, carrots, *garam masala*, coriander powder, cumin powder and salt. Mix.
10. Add water and lemon juice.
11. Mix and bring water to a boil.
12. Reduce heat to low, cover with a tight lid and cook for 30 minutes.
13. Uncover, fluff quinoa gently with a fork, cover and let it rest for 5 minutes.
14. Garnish with cilantro and serve.

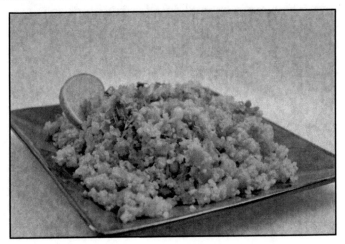

PARATHA – WHOLE WHEAT NORTH INDIAN BREAD

Paratha is an unleavened bread that is an integral part of many Indian meals. It is usually served hot and fresh with a vegetable (*subzi*) or curry dish. Though it requires a little practice, making homemade *paratha* is worth the effort.

Prep Time: 5 minutes plus 15 minutes dough resting time
Cook Time: 15 minutes
Makes: 9

Ingredients:

Whole-wheat flour (Atta) – 1½ cups
Canola oil – 3 tsp
Salt – ¼ tsp (optional)
Warm water – ½ cup + 2 tbsp
Whole-wheat flour (Atta) – ½ cup for dusting and rolling
Canola oil for pan frying

Method:

1. In a large flat bowl, mix flour and salt.
2. Add oil and mix well to incorporate oil into flour.
3. Slowly add warm water and knead to form a dough.
4. Shape dough into a ball and rub a few drops of oil on it to coat.
5. Cover and allow to rest for at least 15 minutes.
6. Knead dough once again. Divide into 9 ping-pong-sized balls.
7. Smoothen each ball in your palms and press into a flat circle.
8. Put ½ cup of whole-wheat flour in flat bowl or dish.
9. Dip the flattened ball into dry flour and coat on all sides.
10. Using a rolling pin, roll out each ball into flat disc – similar to a tortilla.
11. Keep dipping dough into dry flour while rolling so it doesn't stick.
12. Heat a *tawa* or skillet on medium heat.

13. Place the rolled *paratha* on a skillet.
14. When bubbles start to form, flip *paratha* over.
15. After about 10-15 seconds, smear the *paratha* with a little oil and flip over.
16. With a spatula, press *paratha* to make it balloon up.
17. Smear other side with oil and flip over again.
18. Press on bubbles gently to make entire *paratha* balloon.
19. *Paratha* is done when raw dough appears cooked.

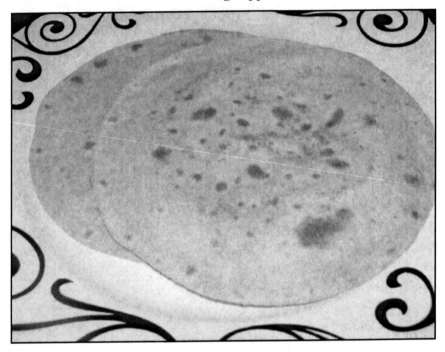

DHEBRA – MILLET AND FENUGREEK FLATBREAD

Dhebra is a unleavened flatbread made with wholemeal millet flour. Fenugreek leaves add an amazing flavor and aroma to this delicious flatbread. With a great shelf life, *dhebra* makes a perfect road trip or on-the-go snack. Make some great *dhebra* memories.

Prep Time: 10 minutes plus 15 minutes dough resting time
Cook Time: 20 minutes
Makes: 7-8

Ingredients:

Whole-wheat flour (Atta) – 1 cup
Millet flour (*bajra*) – ⅓ cup
Yogurt – ½ cup
Citric acid – ¼ tsp (optional if yogurt is not sour)
Jaggery or brown sugar – 1 tbsp
Minced ginger – 2 tsp
Minced garlic – 2 tsp
Sesame seeds – 1 tbsp
Cumin powder – ½ tsp
Turmeric powder – ¼ tsp
Red chili powder – ¼ tsp or to taste
Green chilies – to taste, minced
Salt – 1 tsp or to taste
Dried fenugreek leaves (*kasoori methi*) – 2 tbsp
Cilantro – ¼ cup
Canola oil – 2 tbsp + additional for pan frying

Method:

1. Combine the following – yogurt, citric acid (if being used) and jaggery or brown sugar. Mix well and break any lumps.
2. Add ginger, garlic, sesame seeds, cumin powder, turmeric powder, red chili powder, green chilies, salt, fenugreek leaves

and cilantro. Mix and set aside.

3. To make dough, combine flours and incorporate oil (2 tbsp) into flour.

4. Add yogurt/spice mixture and make dough without using additional water.

5. Knead dough for 3-4 minutes.

6. Drizzle a few drops of oil on dough to coat it, cover and allow it to rest for 15-20 minutes.

7. Heat *tawa* or flat skillet on medium heat.

8. Divide dough into golf-sized balls (approximately 7-8).

9. Form each into a smooth ball and flatten with palms.

10. Dip dough into whole-wheat flour and roll it out using a rolling pin (8-inch). Keep dusting additional flour as needed to prevent sticking.

11. Dust off excess flour and place disc on a hot skillet.

12. Move *dhebra* around so it does not stick. Allow it to cook on one side until a few bubbles appear.

13. Flip the *dhebra* and allow it to cook on the other side.

14. Drizzle a little oil, smear it and flip the *dhebra*.

15. Press down gently but firmly with flat spatula – pressing and rotating.

16. Apply oil on this side, smear, flip and press down again.

17. Remove *dhebra* from skillet and transfer to an insulated container until ready to serve.

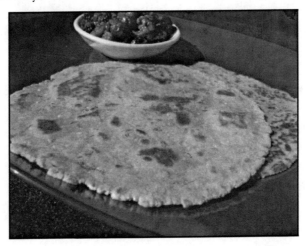

FERMENTED DAIRIES

DAHI – HOMEMADE YOGURT

Ingredients:

Milk – 4 cups
Starter yogurt – 1 heaping tbsp

Method:

1. Bring milk to a boil on the stovetop or in microwave (candy thermometer reading: 180 degrees Fahrenheit).
2. Allow milk to cool down slightly. It should be a little warmer than lukewarm (candy thermometer reading: approx 115 degrees Fahrenheit).
3. Add starter yogurt to milk and mix in with a hand blender or whisk.
4. Transfer milk to a container with a lid.
5. Preheat oven to 180 degrees Fahrenheit and switch oven off.
6. Place container into warm oven and allow the yogurt to set for 3 ½-4 hours.
7. Once set, remove yogurt from oven and store in refrigerator.

Notes:

1. Starter yogurt can be store bought or from previous batch.
2. Do not add the starter into hot milk or the bacteria will die and yogurt will not set.
3. If you prefer tart yogurt, keep the yogurt in warm oven for longer.
4. To make a larger amount, yogurt needs longer time to set.
5. The higher the percentage of fat in the milk, the thicker and denser the yogurt.

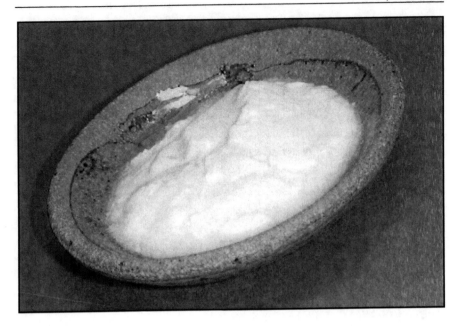

PALAK RAITA – SPINACH IN SPICED YOGURT

Spinach *Raita* is a tasty way to combine two healthy ingredients: spinach and yogurt (*dahi*). Green spinach leaves, loaded with vitamins, are an appetizing contrast to the coolness of the yogurt. *Raita* is an important part of many Indian meals and plays a vital role in helping digestion. Eat this with brown rice or *paratha* or something spicy to help cool down the fire.

Prep Time: 5 minutes
Cook Time: 5 minutes
Serves: 4

Ingredients:

Spinach – 4 cups, chopped
Canola oil – 1 tbsp
Mustard seeds – ½ tsp
Cumin seeds – ½ tsp
Garlic – 3 cloves, finely chopped
Green chili – 1 or to taste, finely chopped
Mint leaves – handful, chopped (cilantro can be substituted)
Yogurt – 2 cups, well beaten
Salt – to taste

Method:

1. Heat oil in a skillet on medium heat.
2. Add mustard seeds and allow them to pop.
3. Add cumin seeds and allow them to sizzle.
4. Add garlic and green chilies. Cook for 1 minute.
5. Add mint leaves and stir.
6. Mix in spinach. Cook for 3-4 minutes.
7. Once spinach wilts, increase heat and allow liquid to evaporate.
8. Remove skillet from heat and cool.
9. Add spinach and salt to yogurt, mix well.

10.   Chill before serving.

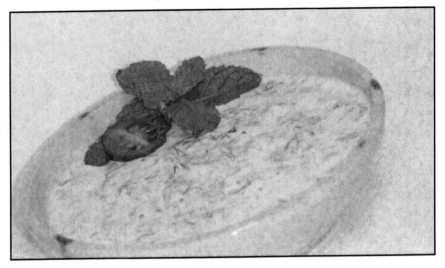

PUDINA LASSI – MINT-FLAVORED YOGURT DRINK

Lassi is a popular yogurt-based drink from Punjab but has gained popularity all over the world for its ability to soothe one's mouth after having had a spicy dish or to cool one down on a hot summer day. *Lassi* comes in many varieties – sweet, salted or fruity. This recipe is a wonderful mint-flavored variation with a kick!

Prep Time: 5 minutes
Serves: 2

Ingredients:

Yogurt – 1 cup
Ice – 1½ cups
Roasted cumin powder – ½ tsp
Chaat masala – 1 tsp
Salt – to taste
Mint – a handful (fresh)
Cilantro – 10 sprigs
Green chili – 1 (optional)

Method:

1. In a blender, add mint, cilantro, green chili and ½ cup yogurt.
2. Blend for a few minutes until smooth.
3. Add remaining ½ cup yogurt and the balance of the ingredients. Blend until the ice is crushed well (smoothie consistency).
4. Serve chilled.

Notes:

1. Dried mint (available at Natural Food Stores) may be substituted for fresh.
2. For a variation, try sweet *lassi*. Use the same proportions of yogurt and ice, add sugar (to taste) and blend until smooth.

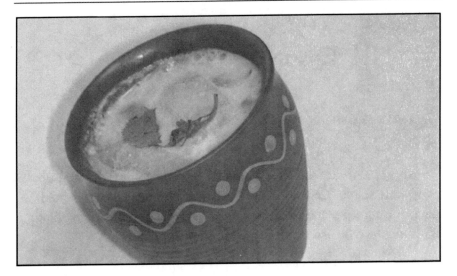

CHUTNEYS AND PICKLES

DHANIYA KI CHUTNEY – CORIANDER (CILANTRO) CHUTNEY

Coriander, also known as *Cilantro*, is a very common and popular garnish in South Asian cooking. Coriander chutney takes this mild, yet flavorful herb and transforms it to a versatile condiment or dipping sauce that can be used with many different appetizers.

Prep Time: 10 minutes

Ingredients:

Cilantro/coriander – 1 big bunch
Jalapenos – 5-6 or to taste
Bell pepper – 1
Chaat masla – ½ tsp
Roasted cumin powder – 1 tsp
Lime/lemon juice – 1 ½ tsp or to taste
Ginger – 1-inch piece
Salt – to taste
Canola oil – 1 tsp

Method:

1. Add all ingredients (except oil) into a blender and grind to a smooth paste.
2. Push down the mixture to help with the grinding process.
3. Add oil right before final whirl to preserve the green color.
4. Store in refrigerator until ready to consume or freeze for longer periods.

COCONUT CHUTNEY

Coconut Chutney is a perfect accompaniment to *dosas*.

Prep time: 15 minutes
Cook time: 20 minutes
Serves: plenty!

Ingredients:

Shredded coconut – 3 cups
Chana dal – ½ cup
Ginger – 2-inch piece
Green chilies – to taste, slit
Cilantro/coriander leaves – small bunch
Curry leaves – 1 sprig
Oil – 1 tbsp
Asafoetida – pinch
Mustard seeds – ½ tsp
Dry red chilies – 1-2
Urad dal – 2 tsp
Salt – to taste
Tamarind pulp – to taste

Method:

1. On medium heat, dry roast *chana dal* until light golden and fragrant.
2. Transfer *dal* into a bowl with water and allow it to soak.
3. Dry roast coconut on medium heat, until light golden and fragrant. Transfer to a blender.
4. Roast ginger and green chilies until light brown. Transfer to blender.
5. Lightly cook cilantro (leaves plus stems) until it wilts. Transfer to blender.
6. Drain *chana dal* and add to blender.

173

7. Add salt and tamarind pulp to taste.
8. Add water and blend to desired consistency.
9. Pour into a serving bowl.
10. Heat oil in a small skillet on medium heat.
11. Add mustard seeds and allow them to pop.
12. Add asafoetida and dry red chilies and cook for 10 seconds.
13. Add *urad dal* and cook until light golden.
14. Add curry leaves, mix and remove from heat.
15. Pour seasoning over chutney.
16. Serve with *dosas*.

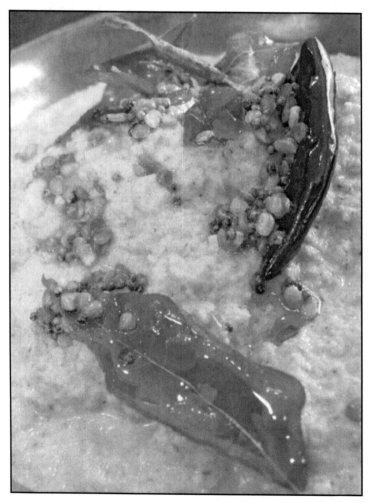

MAANGA AAVAKAI – MANGO PICKLE

Prep Time: 10 minutes
Pickling Time: 20 days

Ingredients:

Raw green mangoes – 2 large (1 lb)
Garbanzo beans, dry (*Kabuli Chana*) – 1 cup
Salt – 1½ tbsp or to taste
Turmeric powder – ¼ tsp
Asafoetida – ¼ tsp
Mustard seed powder – 1 tbsp
Coriander powder – ¼ cup
Red chili powder – 6 tbsp or to taste
Kashmiri chili powder – 1 tbsp
Fenugreek seeds – ¼ tsp, powdered
Sesame seed oil – 1½ cups

Method:

1. Wash and dry mangoes.
2. Remove seed and cube mangoes with a shape knife.
3. Wash and completely dry garbanzo beans.
4. Spread mangoes and garbanzo beans on a tray, cover with thin cloth and allow them to dry overnight.
5. Next day, mix dry spices in a bowl – salt, turmeric, asafoetida, mustard seed powder, coriander powder, red chili powder, *kashmiri* chili powder and fenugreek seed powder.
6. Add mangoes and garbanzo beans. Mix well.
7. Add sesame oil, mix, cover and set bowl out in the sun for about 20 days. Mix daily.
8. Transfer to clean, dry jar and store at room temperature or refrigerator.
9. Enjoy over the next few months.

Tips:

1. Use *kashmiri* chili powder to make a mild pickle.
2. Skip the garbanzo beans and the pickle will be ready in 12 days.
3. Oil should be floating on top to prevent spoilage.

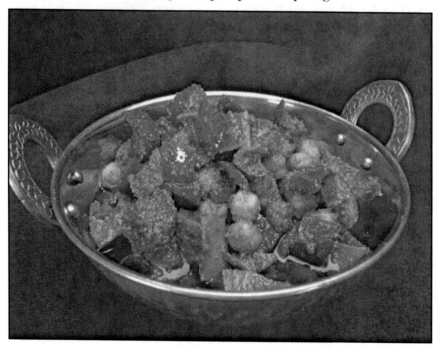

SPICE MIXES

HOMEMADE GARAM MASALA (SPICE POWDER)

Garam masala is a blend of powdered spices that is essential in many Indian recipes. Though store bought, *Garam masala* is convenient, try this recipe and you will understand the impact fresh roasted and ground spices can make to your senses.

Ingredients:

Black cardamom – 12 (10 g)
Coriander seeds – 2 tbsp (10 g)
Cloves – 1 ½ tbsp (10g)
Whole peppercorns – 1 tsp (2½ g)
Cumin seeds – 4 tsp (10 g)
Cinnamon stick – 4-inch piece (10g)
Optional:
Black cumin – 1 tsp
Green cardamom – 2-3 (replace with 1 black cardamom)
Whole peppercorns – to taste (for a spicier *masala*)

Method:

1. Dry roast all ingredients in a heavy-bottomed open skillet on low to medium heat.
2. Stir continuously. Watch for fantastic aroma and a slight change in color.
3. Remove skillet from heat and transfer spices into a plate.
4. Allow spices to cool to room temperature.
5. Break open black cardamom, remove seeds and discard husk.
6. Grind all spices to a fine powder using a coffee or spice grinder.
7. Store *garam masala* in a dry airtight container.
8. Use as required for Indian cooking.

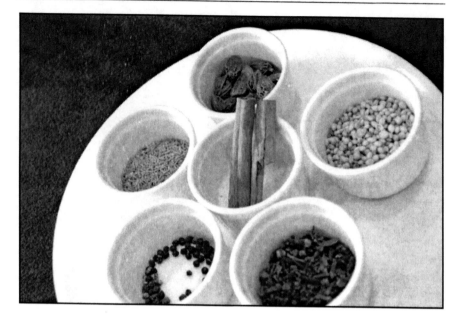

HOMEMADE CURRY POWDER

The Western world has come to rely on curry powder as a convenient one-stop shop in the spice cabinet. With some of the most prominent Indian spices present, curry powder delivers flavor without the fuss.

Ingredients:

Coriander seeds – 2 tbsp
Cumin seeds – 1 tbsp
Fennel seeds – 1 tsp
Mustard seeds – 1 tsp
Black peppercorns – ½ tsp
Turmeric powder – 1 tsp
Red chili powder – ½ tsp
Ginger powder – 1 tsp

Method:

1. Dry roast whole seeds in a heavy-bottomed pan on low heat until lightly golden and fragrant (approximately 10 minutes). Stir continuously.
2. Transfer seeds to a plate and allow them to cool completely.
3. Grind seeds to a fine powder using a spice/coffee grinder.
4. Add remaining powdered spices and mix well.
5. Store in an airtight container in a cool, dry place for up to 3 months.

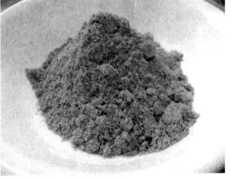

CHAAT (SNACKS) AND SALADS

SHAKARKANDI CHAAT – SWEET POTATO SALAD

Sweet potatoes are a distant relative of white potatoes and commonly marketed as "yams" to differentiate them from the typical potato. Compared with other vegetables, the sweet potato ranks high in complex carbohydrates, dietary fiber, beta-carotene (a precursor to vitamin A), vitamin C, and vitamin B6. Take the sweet potato to a flavor high point with this easy and healthy recipe, and serve this Indian spin on one of nature's nutrient-rich vegetables as an appetizer or side salad.

Prep Time: 5 minutes
Cooking Time: 10 minutes
Serves: 4

Ingredients:

Sweet potatoes – 3 medium (boiled, peeled and chopped)
Cucumber – 1 (peeled and chopped)
Clementine oranges (or any favorite variety) – same amount as cucumber, chopped segments
Salt – to taste
Red chili powder – to taste
Chaat masala – to taste
Lemon/lime juice – to taste
Chopped almonds/walnuts – ¼ cup
Dried cranberries – handful or to taste
Mint leaves – handful, chopped

Method:

1.   Chop sweet potatoes, cucumber and oranges into similar-sized

pieces.
2.   Add all ingredients to a mixing bowl and mix well.
3.   Serve immediately.

If serving later, add lemon/lime juice just before serving to prevent it from becoming dry.

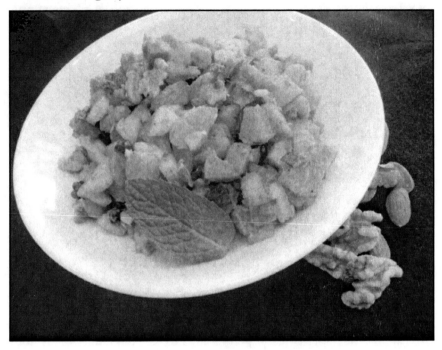

CHUKUNDAR KACHUMBER – BEETROOT SALAD

Beetroot (aka red beets) is a nutrient-rich vegetable that is known for its effects on cardiovascular health and hypertension. Try this simply delicious and colorful beetroot salad recipe that can be a wonderful accompaniment to any meal.

Prep Time: 10 minutes plus 1 hour chilling time (optional)
Serves: 4-6

Ingredients:

Beetroot – 1 lb, peeled and shredded
Roasted peanuts – ½ cup, roughly crushed
Cilantro (coriander) – 5 sprigs, chopped
Green chilies – to taste, finely chopped
Onion – ½ cup, finely chopped
Lemon/lime juice – to taste
Salt – to taste

Method:

Mix all of the ingredients together in a bowl and chill for 1 hour before serving.

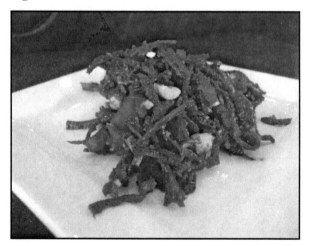

SAMBHARO – COOKED CABBAGE SALAD

Sambharo is a cabbage salad popular in the Indian state of Gujarat. With minimal cooking time, most of the nutrients and vitamin C are still intact. This salad can be enjoyed warm or cold and makes a perfect side dish.

Ingredients:

Cabbage – 6 cups, finely chopped
Carrots – 1 medium, shredded
Canola oil – 1½ tbsp
Mustard seeds – 1 tsp
Asafoetida – ⅛ tsp
Curry leaves – few
Green chilies – 2 or to taste, slit
Salt – to taste
Lemon/lime juice – 1 tbsp
Cilantro – 5 sprigs, finely chopped for garnishing

Method:

1. Heat oil in a medium pan on medium heat.
2. Add mustard seeds and allow them to pop.
3. Add asafoetida, curry leaves, green chilies and cook for approximately 30 seconds.
4. Add lemon/lime juice and salt.
5. Add cabbage and carrots and toss for about 2 minutes.
6. Taste and adjust salt and lemon juice and remove pan from heat.
7. Serve warm, at room temperature or cold.
8. Garnish with cilantro at the time of serving.

Basic Glossary

Atta: Whole-wheat flour made from hard or semi-hard wheat grown on the Indian Subcontinent and used to make *chapatti* and *paratha*.

Curry powder: Mixture of ground spices of widely varying composition based on South Asian cuisines.

Dahi (Yoghurt): Dairy product produced by bacterial fermentation of milk.

Garam masala: Blend of whole spices ground to a fine powder common in South Asian cuisines

Ghee: Clarified butter made by boiling unsalted butter and then straining it to remove any remnant milkfat.

Haldi (Tumeric): A rhizomatous plant of the ginger family native to tropical South Asia that is boiled, dried, and then ground into a deep orange-yellow powder commonly used as a spice in curries for its earthy, slightly bitter and slightly peppery flavor and mustardy smell. Its active ingredient is curcumin.

Maida: Finely milled wheat flour used to make Indian breads such as poori and naan. A.K:A. All-purpose flour or plain flour used for making naan or bhatura.

Pickle: Food made by anaerobic bacterial fermentation of various plant foods in brine or vinegar.

Subzi: Vegetable or dry vegetable preparation.

ACKNOWLEDGEMENTS

This book has been percolating for several years, largely due to the interest and support of my parents, Ramesh and Rajeshree, who used to consistently get on the treadmill and cook healthier Gujarati dishes since I was a kid. My brother Milan's approach to good health was based on whipping up meals from ingredients close to how they're found in nature, and he showed me that fresh plant-based foods, which I knew were healthy, can also taste amazing.

I am grateful to my local papers Indo-American News and India Herald for letting me write on chronic disease. I began studying the scientific literature on the connections between diet and health in earnest after graduating from medical school, thanks mostly to conversations with my college friends Vikrant, Kalyan, and Rajesh. The information and interpretations we sent back and forth since 2008 sparked my search for the truth and ultimately led to this book.

My friends Vineet P. and Ian B. helped shape the direction of these ideas, and the opinions and feedback given me by Stephanie A., Kiran U., Karthik, Shibu, Shreedhar & Ciny, Ketan & Bhavini, Sean S., Soham, Prashant R., Reena P., David G., Jason A., Francis, Dan K., Ankur P., Sonali M., Christina S., Amit M., G.M. Swami, and countless other friends and family I wish I could name, proved extremely valuable. I thank India Currents (California) and Little India (New York) for giving me the opportunity to write articles that organized my thoughts and message on how to make Indian food healthier.

The warm reception my booklet on the Gujarati diet, which I had written for my local temple's health fair, got from friends, family, even strangers, including Mohit & Meeta S., Pravin & Mina P., R.G. Patel, and Jatin P., pushed me to take these ideas from the ether and put them into the word processor. My boss J. Wendt created an environment that encouraged me to push further.

The books and studies I mention in these pages were of the

greatest help, providing the hard evidence supporting the claims I make. It is no exaggeration to say I have stood on the shoulders of giants in the fields where diet, health, and disease intersect. I personally thank R. Thompson and B. Aggarwal among them for conversing with me on their own interests and contributing specifically to this book. I am also thankful for our editor Mark of Angel Editing for giving the book clarity and energy.

Finally, this book would not have seen the light of day were it not for the wonderful chefs Anuja B. and Hetal J., made famous thanks to their enthusiastic demonstrations on YouTube. To discover their desire to share healthy Indian food with the world was both rewarding and a lucky break, and thanks to their understanding of how to make tasty Indian food also good for you, this book is not only a set of ideas but rather a useful guide that people from all walks of life can benefit from.

– Niraj "Raj" R. Patel, M.D.

We would like to thank Raj for giving us the opportunity to be a part of this insightful journey and for providing the science behind our philosophy for healthy cooking.

Our families have been our pillars of support and have willingly put up with "the good, the bad and the tasteless" part of our test kitchen. Their sometimes-ruthless critique has pushed us to keep raising the bar.

We would be nowhere without our loyal viewers. On a daily basis, they lift our spirits, they challenge us, and they teach us. They allow us into their homes and their hearts.

Finally, we'd like to thank Anita for designing the book cover for a project that means a lot to us.

– Hetal Jannu and Anuja Balasubramanian

ENDNOTES

[1] Cruz-Correa, M. et al. "Combination Treatment With Curcumin and Quercetin of Adenomas in Familial Adenomatous Polyposis." Clin Gastroenterology and Hepatology 2006; 4(8):1-4.

[2] Steinbach, G. et al. "The Effect of Celexocib, a Cyclooxygenase-2 Inhibitor, in Familial Adenomatous Polyposis." NEJM 2000; 342(26):1946-1952.

[3] McCarrison, R. "Rice in Relation to Beri-beri in India." Section of Tropical Diseases and Parasitology. Published 3 Mar 1924.

[4] McCarrison, R. "National Health and Nutrition." The Cantor Lectures delivered before The Royal Society of Arts. 1936.

[5] Ibid.

[6] "Obituary notice: Major-General Robert McCarrison, Kt, C.I.E., M.A., M.D., D.Sc., LL.D., F.R.C.P." Brit J Nutr. 1960; 14:413.

[7] Taubes, G. "Good Calories, Bad Calories." Anchor Books, New York: 2007. Pages 98-99.

[8] Taubes, Gary. "Big Fat Lies." Stevens Institute of Technology, Hoboken, New Jersey. 6 February 2008.

[9] Hedley, A.A. et al. "Prevalence of Overweight and Obesity Among US Children, Adolescents, and Adults, 1999-2002." JAMA 2004; 291(23):2847-2850.

[10] Caballero, Benjamin. "The Global Epidemic of Obesity: An Overview." Epidemiol Rev 2007;29(1):1-5.

[11] Thompson, Rob. "Glycemic Load Diet." New York: McGraw Hill, 2006.

[12] Danesh, J. et al. "Chronic infections and coronary heart disease: is there a link?" Lancet 1997; 350(9075): 430-436.

[13] Ornish, D. et al. "Intensive Lifestyle Changes for Reversal of Coronary Heart Disease." JAMA 1998; 280(23):2001-2007.

[14] Ascherio, A. and Willett, W.C. "Health effects of trans fatty acids." Am J Clin Nutr 1997; 66(suppl):1006S-1OS.

[15] Mensink, R.P. "Effects of dietary fatty acids and carbohydrates on the ratio of serum total to HDL cholesterol and on serum lipids and apolipoproteins: a meta-analysis of 60 controlled trials." Amer J Clin Nutr 2003; 77(5):1146-1155.

[16] Accurso, A. et al. "Dietary carbohydrate restriction in type 2 diabetes mellitus and metabolic syndrome: time for a critical appraisal." Nutrition & Metabolism 2008; 5:9.

[17] Boden, G. "Effect of a Low-Carbohydrate Diet on Appetite, Blood Glucose Levels, and Insulin Resistance in Obese Patients with Type 2 Diabetes." Ann of Int Med 2005; 142(6):403-411.

[18] "Metabolic Syndrome." Hosted by American Heart Association. URL: http://www.americanheart.org/presenter.jhtml?identifier=4756. Accessed by 12 Feb 2011.

[19] Yamashita, S. et al. "Insulin resistance and body fat distribution." Diabetes Care 1996; 19(3):287-291.

[20] Banerjee, M.A. et al. "Body Composition, Visceral Fat, Leptin, and Insulin Resistance in Asian Indian Men." JCEM 1999; 84(1):137-144.

[21] Grundy, S.M. "Obesity, Metabolic Syndrome, and Cardiovascular Disease." JCEM 2004; 89(6):2595-2600.

[22] JAMA patient page: the metabolic syndrome.

[23] Soto, A.M. and Sonnenschein, C. "Environmental causes of cancer: endocrine disruptors as carcinogens." Nature Reviews Endocrinology 2010; 6:363-370.

[24] Anand, P. et al. "Cancer is a Preventable Disease that Requires Major Lifestyle Changes." Pharm Res. 2008; 25(9):2097–2116.

[25] "Cancer." World Health Organization. URL: http://www.who.int/mediacentre/factsheets/fs297/en, Updated Feb 2009. Accessed Dec 2010.

[26] Ornish, D. et al. "Intensive lifestyle changes may affect the progression of prostate cancer." Journal of Urology 2005; 174:1065-1070.

[27] Dvorak, Harold F. "Tumors: Wounds That Do Not Heal." N Engl J Med 1986; 315:1650-1659.

[28] Peek, Richard M. et al. "Inflammation in the Genesis and Perpetuation of Cancer: Summary and Recommendations from a National Cancer Institute–Sponsored Meeting." Cancer Res October 1, 2005 65; 8583.

[29] Marx, J. "Inflammation and Cancer: The Link Grows Stronger." Science 2004; 306(5698):966-968.

[30] Servan-Schreiber, D. "Anticancer." Penguin Group: New York, 2009.

[31] Rothwell, Peter M. "Effect of daily aspirin on long-term risk of death due to cancer: analysis of individual patient data from randomised trials." The Lancet, Early Online Publication, 7 December 2010.

[32] Gilmore, T.D. "Introduction to NF-$\varkappa$B: players, pathways, perspectives." Oncogene 2006; 25:6680–6684.

[33] Colotta, F. and Mantovani, A. "Targeted therapies in cancer: myth or reality?" Springer Science + Business Media: New York, 2008.

[34] Singh, S. and Aggarwal, B.B. "Activation of transcription factor NF-kappa B is suppressed by curcumin (diferuloylmethane)." J Biol Chem. 1995;270(42):24995-25000.

[35] Bray, G.A. "Medical consequences of obesity." J Clin Endo Met 2004; 89(6):2583-2589.

[36] "Obesity and cancer: questions and answers." National Cancer Institute. URL: http://www.cancer.gov/cancertopics/factsheet/Risk/obesity. Accessed 13 Jan 2011.

[37] Hokanson, J.E. and Austin, M.A. "Plasma triglyceride level is a risk factor for cardiovascular disease independent of high-density lipoprotein cholesterol level: a meta-analysis of population-based prospective studies." Journal of Cardiovascular Risk 1996; 3(2):213-219.

[38] Wisee, B.E. "The inflammatory syndrome: the role of adipose tissue cytokines in metabolic disorders linked to obesity." J Am Soc Nephrol 2004; 15:2792-2800.

[39] Forsythe, Cassandra E. et al. "Comparison of Low Fat and Low Carbohydrate Diets on Circulating Fatty Acid Composition and Markers of Inflammation." Lipids (2008) 43:65–77.

[40] Taubes, G. "Good Calories, Bad Calories." Anchor Books, New York: 2007. Pages 102-103, 115-116.

[41] "National Diabetes Statistics, 2007." Hosted by National Institutes of Health. URL: http://www.diabetes.niddk.nih.gov/dm/pubs/statistics. Updated Jun 2008. Accessed 3 Feb 2011.

[42] Cleave, T.L. "The Saccharine Disease." Bristol: John Wright & Sons, Ltd. 1974.

[43] Caballero, B. "A Nutrition Paradox — Underweight and Obesity in Developing Countries." N Engl J Med 2005; 352:1514-1516.

[44] Ball, J. "Dr. Oz: Make Meditation Your New Year's Resolution." David Lynch Foundation, New York. 13 December 2010.

[45] Taubes, G. "Good Calories, Bad Calories." Anchor Books: New York, 2008. Pages 335-356.

[46] Pirozzo, S. et al. "Advice on low-fat diets for obesity." Cochrane Database Syst Rev 2002; 2:CD003640.

[47] Yancy, W.S. et al. "A Low-Carbohydrate, Ketogenic Diet versus a Low-Fat Diet To Treat Obesity and Hyperlipidemia." Ann Int Med 2004; 140(10):769-777.

[48] Siri-Tarino, P.W. et al. "Meta-analysis of prospective cohort studies evaluating the association of saturated fat with cardiovascular disease." Am J Clin Nutr 2010; 91(3):535-546.

[49] Sarwar, N. et al. "Triglycerides and the Risk of Coronary Heart Disease." Circulation 2007; 115:450-458.

[50] Yancy, W.S. et al. "A Low-Carbohydrate, Ketogenic Diet versus a Low-Fat Diet To Treat Obesity and Hyperlipidemia." Ann of Int Med 2004; 140(10):769-777.

[51] Jameson, Marni. "A reversal on carbs: Fat was once the devil. Now more nutritionists are pointing accusingly at sugar and refined grains." Los Angeles Times. 20 December 2010. (Accessed 20 December 2010.)

[52] Willett, Walter C. and Skerrett, Patrick J. "Eat, Drink, and Be Healthy." Free Press: New York, 2001. Pages 54-55.

[53] Volek, Jeff S. et al. "Carbohydrate Restriction has a More Favorable Impact on the Metabolic Syndrome than a Low Fat Diet." Lipids (2009) 44:297–309.

[54] Hu, F.B. and Willett, W.C. "Optimal Diets for Prevention of Coronary Heart Disease." JAMA 2002; 288(20):2569-2578.

[55] Siri-Tarino, P.W. et al. "Meta-analysis of prospective cohort studies evaluating the association of saturated fat with cardiovascular disease." Am J Clin Nutr 2010; 91(3):535-46.

[56] Prior, I.A. et al. "Cholesterol, coconuts, and diet on Polynesian atolls: a natural experiment: the Pukapuka and Tokelau island studies." Am J Clin Nutr 1981; 34(8):1552-61.

[57] Mozaffarian, D., Rimm, E.B., and Herrington, D.M. "Dietary fats, carbohydrate, and progression of coronary atherosclerosis in postmenopausal women." Am J Clin Nutr 2004; 80(5):1175-1184.

[58] Malhotra, S.L. "Epidemiology of Ischaemic Heart Disease in India with Special Reference to Causation." Brit Heart J 1967; 29:895-905.

[59] Mente, A. "A Systematic Review of the Evidence Supporting a Causal Link Between Dietary Factors and Coronary Heart Disease." Arch Intern Med. 2009; 169(7):659-669.

[60] Norton A. Study fails to link saturated fat, heart disease. Reuters.

[61] "Fats and Cholesterol: Out with the Bad, In with the Good." Harvard School of Public Health. URL: http://www.hsph.harvard.edu/nutritionsource/what-should-you-eat/fats-full-story/index.html#cholesterol. Accessed 15 Jan 2011.

[62] "Omega-3 Fatty Acids: An Essential Contribution." Hosted by Harvard School of Public Health. URL: http://www.hsph.harvard.edu/nutritionsource/what-should-you-eat/omega-3-fats/index.html. Accessed 12 Feb 2011.

[63] Jakobsen, M.U. et al. "Major types of dietary fat and risk of coronary heart disease: a pooled analysis of 11 cohort studies." Am J Clin Nutr 2009; 89(5):1425-1432.

[64] Simopoulos, A.P. "Essential fatty acids in health and chronic disease." Am J Clin Nutr 1999; 70(3):560S-569S.

[65] Richard, D. et al. "Polyunsaturated fatty acids as antioxidants." Pharmacological Research 2008; 57(6):451-455.

[66] "Is it OK to cook with extra-virgin olive oil?" The George Mateljan Foundation. URL: http://www.whfoods.com/genpage.php?tname=george&dbid=56. Accessed 7 Jan 2010.

[67] "Fats and Cholesterol: Out with the Bad, In with the Good." Harvard School of Public Health. URL: http://www.hsph.harvard.edu/nutritionsource/what-should-you-eat/fats-full-story/index.html#cholesterol. Accessed 15 Jan 2011.

[68] Taubes, G. "Good Calories, Bad Calories." Anchor Books, New York: 2007. Page 200.

[69] Saturated fat, carbohydrate, and cardiovascular disease. ACJN 2010.

[70] Atkinson, F.S., Foster-Powel, K., and Brand-Miller, J.C. "International Tables of Glycemic Index and Glycemic Load Values: 2008." Diabetes Care 2008; 31:2281-2283.

[71] Salmerón J. et al. "Dietary Fiber, Glycemic Load, and Risk of Non—insulin-dependent Diabetes Mellitus in Women." JAMA 1997; 277(6):472-477.

[72] Chandalia, M. et al. "Beneficial effects of high dietary fiber intake in patiens with type 2 diabetes mellitus." N Engl J Med 2000; 342:1392-8.

[73] "Short chain fatty acids." Institute Danone. URL: http://web.archive.org/web/20071019191020/www.danone-institute.be/communication/pdf/mono03/mono3-part4.pdf. Accessed 3 Jan 2011.

[74] Rimm, E.B. et al. "Vegetable, Fruit, and Cereal Fiber Intake and Risk of Coronary Heart Disease Among Men." JAMA 1996; 275(6):447-451.

[75] Meyer, K.A. et al. "Carbohydrates, dietary fiber, and incident type 2 diabetes in older women." Am J Clin Nutr 2000; 71:921–30.

[76] "Protein: Moving Closer to Center Stage." Hosted by Harvard School of Public Health. URL: http://www.hsph.harvard.edu/nutritionsource/what-should-you-eat/protein-full-story/index.html. Accessed 4 Feb 2011.

[77] Mangels, R. "Protein in the Vegan Diet." Hosted by The Vegetarian Resource Group. URL: http://www.vrg.org/nutrition/protein.htm. Accessed 3 Feb 2011.

[78] Cross, A.J. et al. "A Prospective Study of Red and Processed Meat Intake in Relation to Cancer Risk." PLoS Med 2007; 4(12):e325.

[79] Stanner, S.A. et al. "A review of the epidemiological evidence for the 'antioxidant hypothesis'" Public Health Nutrition 2003; 7(3):407–422.

[80] Gann, P.H. et al. "Lower Prostate Cancer Risk in Men with Elevated Plasma Lycopene Levels." Cancer Res 1999; 59:1225.

[81] Park Y, Hunter DJ, Spiegelman D, et al. "Dietary Fiber Intake and Risk of Colorectal Cancer: A Pooled Analysis of Prospective Cohort Studies." JAMA 2005; 294:2849–2857.

[82] Fraser, G.E. "Vegetarian diets: what do we know of their effects on common chronic diseases?" Am J Clin Nutr 2009; 89(5):1607S-1612S.

[83] "NIH State-of-the-Science Panel Urges More Informed Approach to Multivitamin/Mineral Use for Chronic Disease Prevention." NIH Office of the Director. Published 17 May 2006. Accessed 14 Jan 2011.

[84] de Lorgeril, M. et al. "Mediterranean Diet, Traditional Risk Factors, and the Rate of Cardiovascular Complications After Myocardial Infarction." Circulation 1999; 99:779-785.

[85] Scarmeas, N. et al. "Mediterranean diet and Alzheimer disease mortality." Neurology 200; 69(11):1084–1093.

[86] "Mediterranean Diet." American Heart Association. URL: http://www.americanheart.org/presenter.jhtml?identifier=4644. Accessed 14 Jan 2011.

[87] Masala, G. et al. "A dietary pattern rich in olive oil and raw vegetables is associated with lower mortality in Italian elderly subjects." British Journal of Nutrition 2007; 98:406-415.

[88] Menotti, A. et al. "Food intake patterns and 25-year mortality from coronary heart disease: cross-cultural correlations in the Seven Countries Study. The Seven Countries Study Research Group." Eur J Epidemiol 1999; 15(6):507-15.

[89] "Vegetarian eating." American Dietetic Association. Accessed 16 Jan 2011.

[90] "ADA position paper on vegetarianism." American Dietetic Association. Hosted by the Vegan Resource Group. Accessed 16 Jan 2011.

[91] American Dietetic Association. "ADA position paper on vegetarianism." Hosted by the Vegan Resource Group.

[92] Food and Nutrition Board, Institute of Medicine. "Dietary Reference Intakes for Energy, Carbohydrate, Fiber, Fat, Fatty Acids, Cholesterol, Protein, and Amino Acids." Washington, DC: National Academy Press, 2002.

[93] "Protein in the vegan diet." The Vegetarian Resource Group. URL: http://www.vrg.org/nutrition/protein.htm. Accessed 16 Jan 2011.

[94] Sellmeyer, D.E. et al."A high ratio of dietary animal to vegetable protein increases the rate of bone loss and the risk of fracture in postmenopausal women. Study of Osteoporotic Fractures Research Group." Am J Clin Nutr 2001; 73(1):118-22.

[95] Knight, E.L. et al. "The impact of protein intake on renal function decline in women with normal renal function or mild renal insufficiency." Ann Intern Med 2003; 138(6):460-7.

[96] Cross, A.J. et al. "A Prospective Study of Red and Processed Meat Intake in Relation to Cancer Risk." PLoS Med 2007; 4(12):e325.

[97] "The China Study." URL: http://www.thechinastudy.com. Accessed 10 Jan 2011.

[98] "Prevent and Reverse Heart Disease." URL: http://www.heartattackproof.com. Accessed 10 Jan 2011.

[99] Mangels, R. "Calcium in the vegan diet." Vegan Resource Group. Published 28 Mar 2006. Accessed 19 Jan 2011.

[100] Liu, S. et al. "Intake of vegetables rich in carotenoids and risk of coronary heart disease in men: The Physicians' Health Study." Int. J. Epidemiol. 2001; 30(1):130-135.

[101] Chan J.M. et al. "Diet after diagnosis and the risk of prostate cancer progression, recurrence, and death (United States)." Cancer Causes Control 2006; 17(2):199-208.

[102] Beattie, J. et al. "Potential Health Benefits of Berries." Current Nutrition & Food Science 2005; 1:71-86.

[103] Vizzotto, Marcia. "Inhibition of invasive breast cancer cell growth by selected peach and plum phenolic antioxidants." Thesis. Texas A&M University, College Station: 2005.

[104] Pantuck, A.J. et al. "Phase II Study of Pomegranate Juice for Men with Rising Prostate-Specific Antigen following Surgery or Radiation for Prostate Cancer." Clin Cancer Res 2006; 12:4018.

[105] Nigam, N. et al. "Lupeol induces p53 and cyclin-B-mediated G2/M arrest and targets apoptosis through activation of caspase in mouse skin." Biochem Biophys Res Comm 2009; 381(2):253-258.

[106] Dan Buettner. "Longevity, the Secrets of Long Life." National Geographic magazine. Published Nov 2005.

[107] Seventh-Day Adventist Dietetic Association. "The Seventh-day Adventist Position Statement on Vegetarian Diets." URL: http://www.sdada.org/position.htm. Accessed 19 Jan 2011.

[108] Chandra, V. et al. "Prevalence of Alzheimer's disease and other dernentias in rural India." Neurology 1998; 51:1000-1008.

[109] Bazzano, L.A. et al. "Dietary Fiber Intake and Reduced Risk of Coronary Heart Disease in US Men and Women." Arch Intern Med 2003; 163:1897-1904.

[110] "Fiber." Published by UWSP University Health Service on Sep 2002. URL: http://wellness.uwsp.edu/medinfo/handouts/LAs/Fiber.pdf. Accessed 19 Jan 2011.

[111] Woods, K.L. et al. "Intravenous magnesium sulphate in suspected acute myocardial infarction: results of the second Leicester Intravenous Magnesium Intervention Trial (LIMIT-2)." Lancet 1992; 339(8809):1553-1558.

[112] "Dal." Published by Wikipedia. URL: http://en.wikipedia.org/wiki/Dal. Accessed 19 Jan 2011.

[113] Pittaway, J.K. et al. "Dietary supplementation with chickpeas for at least 5 weeks results in small but significant reductions in serum total and low-density lipoprotein cholesterols in adult women and men." Ann Nutr Metab 2006; 50(6):512-8.

[114] "Garbanzo beans." The George Mateljan Foundation. URL: http://www.whfoods.com/genpage.php?tname=foodspice&dbid=58. Accessed 19 Jan 2010.

[115] Aggarwal, B. et al. "Curcumin – The Indian Solid Gold." URL: http://www.curcuminresearch.org. Accessed 19 Jan 2011.

[116] Duatre, V.M. et al. "Curcumin Enhances the Effect of Cisplatin in Suppression of Head and Neck Squamous Cell Carcinoma via Inhibition of IKKβ Protein of the NFκB Pathway." Mol Cancer Ther 2010; 9:2665.

[117] Lin, Y.G. et al. "Curcumin Inhibits Tumor Growth and Angiogenesis in Ovarian Carcinoma by Targeting the Nuclear Factor-κB Pathway." Clin Cancer Res 2007; 13:3423.

[118] Barnes, P.J. and Karin, M. "Nuclear Factor-κB — A Pivotal Transcription Factor in Chronic Inflammatory Diseases." N Engl J Med 1997; 336:1066-1071.

[119] Escárcega, R.O. et al. "The Transcription Factor Nuclear Factor-kappa B and Cancer." Clinical Oncology 2007; 19(2):154-161.

[120] Chandra, V. et al. "Incidence of Alzheimer's disease in a rural community in India: the Indo-US study." Neurology 2001; 57(6):985-9.

[121] Andersen, K. et al. "Do nonsteroidal anti-inflammatory drugs decrease the risk for Alzheimer's disease? The Rotterdam Study." Neurology 1995; 45(8):1441-5.

[122] Ringman, J.M. et al. "A Potential Role of the Curry Spice Curcumin in Alzheimer's Disease." Curr Alzheimer Res 2005; 2(2):131-136.

[123] Soni, K.B. and Kuttan, R. "Effect of oral curcumin administration on serum peroxides and cholesterol levels in human volunteers." Indian J Physiol Pharmacol 1992; 36(4):273-275.

[124] Shoba, G. et al. "Influence of Piperine on the Pharmacokinetics of Curcumin in Animals and Human Volunteers." Planta Med 1998; 64(4):353-356.

[125] McNamara, F.N., Randall, A., and Gunthorpe, M.J. "Effects of piperine, the pungent component of black pepper, at the human vanilloid receptor (TRPV1)." Br J Pharmacol 2005; 144(6):781-790.

[126] Rahman, K. and Lowe, G.M. "Garlic and Cardiovascular Disease: A Critical Review." J Nutr 2006;136:736S-740S.

[127] Altman, R. D. and Marcussen, K. C. "Effects of a ginger extract on knee pain in patients with osteoarthritis." Arthritis & Rheumatism 2001; 44(11):2531-2538.

[128] Grzanna, R., Lindmark, L. and Frondoza, C.G. "Ginger—An Herbal Medicinal Product with Broad Anti-Inflammatory Actions." J Med Food 2005; 8(2):125-132.

[129] Ahujaa, K.D.K. and Ball, M.J. "Effects of daily ingestion of chilli on serum lipoprotein oxidation in adult men and women." Brit J Nutr 2006; 96:239-242.

[130] Mori, A. et al. "Capsaicin, a Component of Red Peppers, Inhibits the Growth of Androgen-Independent, p53 Mutant Prostate Cancer Cells." Cancer Res 2006; 66:3222.

[131] Khan, A. et al. "Cinnamon Improves Glucose and Lipids of People With Type 2 Diabetes." Diabetes Care 2003; 26:3215-3218.

[132] Altschuler, J.A. et al. "The Effect of Cinnamon on A1C Among Adolescents With Type 1 Diabetes." Diabetes Care 2007; 30(4):813-816.

[133] Vanschoonbeek, K. et al. "Cinnamon Supplementation Does Not Improve Glycemic Control in Postmenopausal Type 2 Diabetes Patients." J Nutr 2006; 136:977-980.

[134] Gray, A.M. and Flatt, P.R. "Insulin-releasing and insulin-like activity of the traditional anti-diabetic plant Coriandrum sativum (coriander)." Brit J Nutr 1999; 81:203-209.

[135] Chithra, V. and Leelamma, S. "Hypolipidemic effect of coriander seeds (Coriandrum sativum): mechanism of action." Plant Foods for Human Nutrition 1997; 51(2):167-172.

[136] Milan, K.S.M. et al. "Enhancement of digestive enzymatic activity by cumin (Cuminum cyminum L.) and role of spent cumin as a bionutrient." Food Chemistry 2008; 110(3):678-683.

[137] Srivastava, K.C. "Extracts from two frequently consumed spices – Cumin (Cuminum cyminum) and turmeric (Curcuma longa) – Inhibit platelet aggregation and alter eicosanoid biosynthesis in human blood platelets." Prostaglandins, Leukotrienes and Essential Fatty Acids 1989; 37(1):57-64.

[138] Agarwal, K.N. and Bhasin, S.K. "Feasibility studies to control acute diarrhoea in children by feeding fermented milk preparations Actimel and Indian Dahi." Eur J Clin Nutr. 2002 Dec;56 Suppl 4:S56-9.

[139] Wollowski, I. et al. "Protective role of probiotics and prebiotics in colon cancer." Amer J of Clin Nut 2001; 73(2):451S-455s.

[140] Larsson, S.C. et al. "High-fat dairy food and conjugated linoleic acid intakes in relation to colorectal cancer incidence in the Swedish Mammography Cohort." Amer J Clin Nut 2005; 82(4):894-900.

[141] Meyer, A.L. et al. "Daily intake of probiotic as well as conventional yogurt has a stimulating effect on cellular immunity in young healthy women." Ann Nutr Metab. 2006; 50(3):282-9.

[142] Gill, H.S. et al. "Enhancement of immunity in the elderly by dietary supplementation with the probiotic Bifidobacterium lactis HN019." Amer J Clin Nut 2001; 74(6): 833-839.

[143] Zemel, M.B. et al. "Dairy augmentation of total and central fat loss in obese subjects." Int J Obesity 2005; 29:391-397.

[144] Skinner, J.D. et al. "Longitudinal calcium intake is negatively related to children's body fat indexes." J Am Diet Assoc. 2003 Dec;103(12):1626-31.

[145] Lin, Y.C. et al. "Dairy Calcium is Related to Changes in Body Composition during a Two-Year Exercise Intervention in Young Women." J Amer Coll Nutr 2000; 19(6):754-760.

[146] Pereira, M.A. et al. "Dairy Consumption, Obesity, and the Insulin Resistance Syndrome in Young Adults." JAMA 2002; 287(16):2081-2089.

[147] Zemel, M.B. "Role of calcium and dairy products in energy partitioning and weight management." Amer J Clin Nutr 2004; 79(5): 907S-912S.

[148] Sun, Q. et al. "White Rice, Brown Rice, and Risk of Type 2 Diabetes in US Men and Women." Arch Intern Med 2010; 170(11):961-969.

[149] de Munter, J.S.L. et al. "Whole Grain, Bran, and Germ Intake and Risk of Type 2 Diabetes: A Prospective Cohort Study and Systematic Review." PLoS Med 4(8): e261.

[150] Lichtenstein, A.H. et al. "Diet and Lifestyle Recommendations Revision 2006." Circulation 2006; 114:82-96.

[151] Koh-Banerjee, P. et al. "Changes in whole-grain, bran, and cereal fiber consumption in relation to 8-y weight gain among men." Am J Clin Nutr 2004; 80(5):1237-1245.

[152] Schatzkin, A. et al. "Dietary fiber and whole-grain consumption in relation to colorectal cancer in the NIH-AARP Diet and Health Study." Amer J Clin Nutr 2007; 85(5):1353-1360.

[153] Sinha, R. et al. "Cancer Risk and Diet in India." J Postgrad Med 2003;49:222-228.

[154] Shakar, S.R. et al. "Serum lipid response to introducing ghee as a partial placement for mustard oil in the diet of healthy young Indians." Indian J Physiol Pharmacol 2005; 49(1):49–56.

[155] "What are the advantages and disadvantages of butter and ghee when it comes to cooking?" The George Mateljan Foundation. URL: http://www.whfoods.com/genpage.php?tname=newtip&dbid=9. Accessed 21 December 2010.

[156] Musarra, Gian. "Breaking Down Baby Formula." St. Louis Children's Hospital. URL: http://www.stlouischildrens.org/content/healthinfo/breakingdownbabyformula.htm. Accessed 21 December 2010.

[157] Manore, Melinda, Nanna Meyer and Janice Thompson. "Sport Nutrition for Health and Performance." 2nd ed. Champaugn, Illinois: Human Kinetics, 2009.

[158] Hobson, Katherine. "Do Coconut Oil and Coconut Water Provide Health Benefits?" U.S. News and World Report. 10 August 2009.

[159] Stanhope, John M. et al. "The Tokelau island migrant study: Serum lipid concentrations in two environments." Journal of Chronic Diseases 1981; 34:45-55.

[160] Prior, I.A. et al. "Cholesterol, coconuts, and diet on Polynesian atolls: a natural experiment: the Pukapuka and Tokelau island studies." American Journal of Clinical Nutrition 1981; 34:1552-1561.

[161] German, B. and Dillard, C.J. "Saturated fats: what dietary intake?" Amer J Clin Nutr 2004; 80(3):550-559.

[162] Fife, B. "The Coconut Oil Miracle." Penguin Group: New York, 2004. Page 12.

[163] Wolke, Robert L. "Canola Baloney." Washington Post. 7 February 2001.

[164] Kontogianni, Meropi D. et al. "The impact of olive oil consumption pattern on the risk of acute coronary syndromes: the cardio2000 case–control study." Clinical Cardiology March 2007; 30(3):125–129.

[165] Psaltopoulou, T. "Olive oil, the Mediterranean diet, and arterial blood pressure: the Greek European Prospective Investigation into Cancer and Nutrition (EPIC) study." Am J Clin Nutr. 2004 Oct;80(4):1012-8.

[166] "Erucic acid in food." Food Standards Australia New Zealand. URL: http://www.foodstandards.gov.au/_srcfiles/Erucic%20acid%20monograph.pdf. Published June 2003. Accessed 11 Jan 2010.

[167] Rastogi, T. et al. "Diet and risk of ischemic heart disease in India." Amer J Clin Nutr 2005; 79(4):582-592.

[168] Harris, W.S. et al. "Omega-6 fatty acids and risk for cardiovascular disease." Circulation 2009; 119:902-907.

[169] Mozaffarian, D. et al. "Trans Fatty Acids and Cardiovascular Disease." N Engl J Med 2006; 354:1601-1613.

[170] Acherio, A. et al. "Trans-Fatty Acids Intake and Risk of Myocardial Infarction." Circulation 1994; 89:94-101.)

[171] Sabaté, Joan et al. "Nut Consumption and Blood Lipid Levels: A Pooled Analysis of 25 Intervention Trials." Arch Intern Med. 2010;170(9):821-827.

[172] Fraser, G.E. et al. "A possible protective effect of nut consumption on risk of coronary heart disease. The Adventist Health Study." Arch Intern Med. 1992 Jul;152(7):1416-24.

[173] Hu, F.B. et al. "Frequent nut consumption and risk of coronary heart disease in women: prospective cohort study." BMJ. 1998 Nov 14;317(7169):1341-5.

[174] Kris-Etherton P.M. et al. "The role of tree nuts and peanuts in the prevention of coronary heart disease: multiple potential mechanisms." J Nutr. 2008 Sep;138(9):1746S-1751S.

[175] Calder, Philip C. "n–3 Polyunsaturated fatty acids, inflammation, and inflammatory diseases." Am J Clin Nutr June 2006 vol. 83 no. 6 S1505-1519S.

[176] Simopoulos, Artemis P. "Omega-3 Fatty Acids in Inflammation and Autoimmune Diseases." J Ame Coll Nutr. 2002; 21(6): 495-505.

[177] Kris-Etherton, P.M. et al. "Fish Consumption, Fish Oil, Omega-3 Fatty Acids, and Cardiovascular Disease." Arteriosclerosis, Thrombosis, and Vascular Biology. 2003;23:e20-e30.

[178] "Omega-3 fatty acids." The George Mateljan Foundation. URL: http://www.whfoods.com/genpage.php?tname=nutrient&dbid=84. Accessed 29 December 2010.

[179] Thompson, Rob. "The Glycemic-Load Diet." McGraw-Hill: New York, 2006. Pages 70-73.

[180] Sacks, F.M. et al. "Effects on blood pressure of reduced dietary sodium and the dietary approaches to stop hypertension (DASH) through diet." N Engl J Med 2001; 344:3-10.

[181] Dodani, S. "Excess coronary artery disease risk in South Asian immigrants: Can dysfunctional high-density lipoprotein explain increased risk?" Vasc Health Risk Manag 2008; 4(5):953–961.

[182] "Working Towards Wellness – an Indian perspective." PricewaterhouseCoopers. URL: http://www.pwc.com/en_IN/in/assets/pdfs/india-publication-working-towards-wellness.pdf. Accessed 10 Jan 2010.

[183] Xavier, D. "Treatment and outcomes of acute coronary syndromes in India (CREATE): a prospective analysis of registry data." Lancet 2008; 371(9622):1435-1442.

[184] Gupta, M. et al. "South Asians and Cardiovascular Risk: What Clinicians Should Know." Circulation 2006; 113:e924-e929.

[185] Kathiresan, S."Lp(a) Lipoprotein Redux — From Curious Molecule to Causal Risk Factor." N Engl J Med 2009; 361:2573-2574.

[186] Venkataraman, R. et al. "Prevalence of diabetes mellitus and related conditions in Asian Indians living in the United States." Amer J Cardiology 2004; 94(7):977-980.

[187] Mindlin, A. "Bedeviled by the Sugar Sickness." New York Times. Published 2 Mar 2008. Accessed 13 Jan 2011.

[188] McKeigue, P.M. et al. "Relation of central obesity and insulin resistance with high diabetes prevalence and cardiovascular risk in South Asians." Lancet 1991; 337(8738):382-386.

[189] Obesity-related non-communicable diseases: South Asians vs White Caucasians.

[190] Ghaffar, A. et al. "Burden of non-communicable diseases in South Asia." BMJ 2004; 328:807-810.

[191] Eapen, D. et al. "Metabolic syndrome and cardiovascular disease in South Asians." Vascular Health and Risk Management 2009; 5:731-743.

[192] Misra, A. "The metabolic syndrome in South Asians." Indian J Med Res 2007; 125:345-354.

[193] Rastogi, T. et al. "Cancer incidence rates among South Asians in four geographic regions: India, Singapore, UK and US." Int J Epidemiol 2008; 37(1):147-160.

[194] Sinha, R. et al. "Cancer Risk and Diet in India." Journal of Postgrad Med 2003; 49(3):222-228.

[195] Misra, A. et al. "Obesity, the Metabolic Syndrome, and Type 2 Diabetes in Developing Countries: Role of Dietary Fats and Oils." J Amer Coll Nutr 2010; 29(3):289S-301S.

[196] Misra, A. et al. "South Asian diets and insulin resistance." Brit J Nutr 2009;101:465-473.

[197] Mohan, V. et al. "Dietary carbohydrates, glycaemic load, food groups and newly detected type 2 diabetes among urban Asian Indian population in Chennai, India." Brit J Nutr 2009; 102:1498-1506.

[198] "Clues Sought for Heart Disease in South Asians." New York Times. Published 9 Aug 1994. Accessed 11 Jan 2011.

CPSIA information can be obtained at www.ICGtesting.com
Printed in the USA
LVOW131718030812

292845LV00011B/123/P